Practical Lambing and Lamb
Care – A Veterinary Guide

Practical Lambing and Lamb Care – A Veterinary Guide

Fourth Edition

Neil Sargison, BA, VetMB, PhD, DSHP, DipECSRHM, FRCVS
University of Edinburgh
Royal (Dick) School of Veterinary Studies
Easter Bush Veterinary Centre
Scotland;
President of the European College of Small Ruminant
Health Management

James Patrick Crilly, MA, VetMB, CertAVP, DipECSRHM, MRCVS
Larkmead Veterinary Group
UK

Andrew Hopker, BVM&S, CertAVP, MRCVS
Royal (Dick) School of Veterinary Studies
Easter Bush Veterinary Centre
Scotland

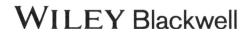
WILEY Blackwell

This edition first published 2018
© 2018 John Wiley & Sons Ltd

Edition History
Longman Group Limited (1st edition, 1986)
Longman Group Limited (2nd edition, 1995)
John Wiley & Sons (3rd edition, 2004)

Registered Office(s)
John Wiley & Sons, Inc., 111 River Street, Hoboken, NJ 07030, USA
John Wiley & Sons Ltd, The Atrium, Southern Gate, Chichester, West Sussex, PO19 8SQ, UK

Editorial Office
9600 Garsington Road, Oxford, OX4 2DQ, UK

For details of our global editorial offices, customer services, and more information about Wiley products visit us at www.wiley.com.

Wiley also publishes its books in a variety of electronic formats and by print-on-demand. Some content that appears in standard print versions of this book may not be available in other formats.

Library of Congress Cataloging-in-Publication Data

Names: Sargison, Neil, author. | Eales, F. A., 1948– Practical lambing and lamb care.
Title: Practical lambing and lamb care / Neil Sargison, University of Edinburgh, Royal (Dick) School of Veterinary Studies, Easter Bush Veterinary Centre, Roslin, Midlothian, James Patrick Crilly, Larkmead Veterinary Group, Ilges Lane, Cholsey, Oxfordshire, Andrew Hopker, Royal (Dick) School of Veterinary Studies, Easter Bush Veterinary Centre, Roslin, Midlothian.
Description: Fourth edition. | Hoboken, NJ : Wiley, 2018. | Revised edition of: Practical lambing and lamb care : a veterinary guide / Andrew Eales and John Small ; with drawings by David Pollock. 3rd ed. 2004. | Includes bibliographical references and index. |
Identifiers: LCCN 2017054875 (print) | LCCN 2017055986 (ebook) | ISBN 9781119133650 (pdf) | ISBN 9781119140672 (epub) | ISBN 9781119140665 (paper)
Subjects: LCSH: Lambs. | Sheep–Parturition. | Veterinary obstetrics. | Lambs–Diseases. | Ewes–Diseases. | Sheep–Diseases.
Classification: LCC SF376.5 (ebook) | LCC SF376.5 .E25 2018 (print) | DDC 636.3/089–dc23
LC record available at https://lccn.loc.gov/2017054875

Cover Design: Wiley
Cover Images: (Top left and bottom images) Courtesy of James Patrick Crilly;
(Top right image) Courtesy of Neil Sargison

Contents

Preface to the Fourth Edition

It has now been fourteen years since the publication of the third edition of *Practical Lambing and Lamb Care*, and 32 years since the first edition. It has been our privilege to update this important globally relevant resource through the preparation of the fourth edition. In doing so, we wish to acknowledge the excellence of the previous editions and the expertise of their Moredun Research Institute-based authors, Colin Macaldowie, John Small, and the sadly missed Andy Eales.

In this new edition, we have attempted to maintain the impressive scope of the previous editions, while focusing on practical husbandry and animal health. We have attempted to extend the scope of the book by including goat kidding management. For clarity, many of the principles referred to under the headings of lambing, ewes and lambs are equally relevant to kidding, goats and kids. The principles of goat management are only described separately where they differ.

We have structured this fourth edition to begin with chapters describing general practical lambing and kidding management, and care of newborn lambs and kids. These chapters describe preparation for lambing or kidding, obstetrical procedures and health management of newborn lambs or kids. Lambing and kidding are part of a management continuum, the outcomes of which are determined by interventions occurring throughout the year. Thus, the foundations for a successful outcome are laid long beforehand. We have dedicated three chapters to animal husbandry and health, describing planned reproductive, nutritional and disease management, with reference to preparation for a successful lambing or kidding. This is followed by a chapter describing a practical approach to ensure that individual sick or unwell animals can be identified and treated promptly. Finally, we have included a chapter describing and explaining animal welfare and disease control legislation.

We are grateful to all of those veterinary colleagues and farmers who have helped us to gain the experience and expertise required in the writing of this book, and to our publisher, Wiley, for their support and patience in this venture.

September 2018   *Neil Sargison*
University of Edinburgh   *James Patrick Crilly*
Royal (Dick) School of Veterinary Studies   *Andrew Hopker*

1

General Lambing Management

It is should be emphasised that most sheep and goats give birth to their lambs and kids naturally and unassisted, as nature intended. When problems do arise, timely intervention is required to prevent losses. However, inappropriate intervention too soon can also cause harm to both ewe and lamb, can compromise animal welfare and may result in economic loss.

The normal hormonal processes involved in giving birth occur most effectively when the dam feels safe and is undisturbed. While good observation is essential, disturbance of the lambing ewes should be minimised and shepherds should move among the flock in a calm and quiet manner. The role of a good shepherd in the delivery of lambs at lambing time should be to provide the right amount of assistance at the right time, and no more. The keys to achieving this are good preparation and adequate supervision of lambing ewes to spot problems in a timely manner.

Most assisted deliveries can be undertaken satisfactorily, using a gentle hygienic technique to give a viable, humane and profitable outcome. The general principles and practice of delivering goat kids are the same as those for lambing ewes. In this chapter, specific reference to goats is only made where the important principles differ.

Preparation for Lambing

Around the world, the economics of small ruminant farming have necessitated a shift of focus away from the care of individual animals and towards whole flock or herd approaches. Careful preparation for lambing or kidding is now, therefore, of paramount importance to protect of the welfare of pregnant and lambing ewes or does, and their newborn lambs or kids. Lambing should be seen as the critical time when the benefits of general preparation, nutrition and animal health management throughout the year are realised.

Careful shepherding and the design and selection of the lambing environment – be it in lambing paddocks, or lambing sheds – is required to minimise disturbance of lambing ewes, thus enabling the establishment of a good ewe-lamb bond and enhancing the survival of newborn lambs. Whenever possible, steep

Practical Lambing and Lamb Care – A Veterinary Guide, Fourth Edition.
Neil Sargison, James Patrick Crilly and Andrew Hopker.
© 2018 John Wiley & Sons Ltd. Published 2018 by John Wiley & Sons Ltd.

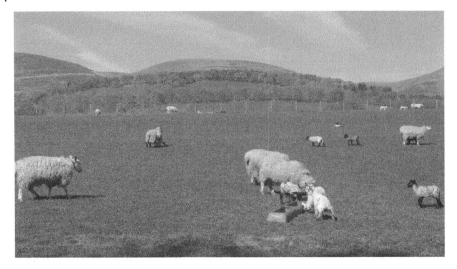

Figure 1.1 Lambing fields should ideally be small and flat with easy access to food and water.

and exposed fields should be avoided. Lambing fields should not be too large and water sources not too far apart (Figure 1.1).

When potentially less suitable lambing paddocks must be used, they should, if possible, be reserved for single-bearing adult ewes. Buildings should be well ventilated and drained. Pens should be small enough to allow animals to be grouped according to their nutritional and animal health needs, and should be designed in a manner such that lambing and lambed ewes can be isolated and removed without undue disturbance of the whole group. Consideration should be given to the housed ewe space requirements of about $1.1\,\mathrm{m}^2$ per ewe, the need for constant access to forage, and concentrate feed trough space requirements of about $0.5\,\mathrm{m}$ per ewe (Figure 1.2). These requirements vary with breed and litter size.

Sufficient individual pens should be available, based on a figure of about 10% for the flock. These should be large enough to allow the ewe and lamb to lie safely apart from each other, and need to be clean and well drained. All pens should be well lit and easily accessible. Food and water must be available at all times.

Despite long-term planning, the need for careful skilled assistance for some lambing ewes is inevitable. A clear plan is required to avoid suffering in ewes which cannot be lambed. This should include guidelines about when and how to seek assistance and provision for the immediate humane destruction of distressed animals. Lambing equipment should be prepared in advance (see Table 1.1). Provision should be made for the management of those diseases which occur annually in most flocks around lambing, and there should also be clear guidelines about when to seek assistance, and to ensure prompt and humane destruction to prevent further suffering when treatment is unsuccessful or uneconomical. Preparation for lambing must also be aimed at prevention and management of disease in newborn lambs. Despite careful preventive management, the occurrence of disease in newborn lambs is inevitable, so provision should be made for the treatment of the common problems and specific diseases that occur in the flock.

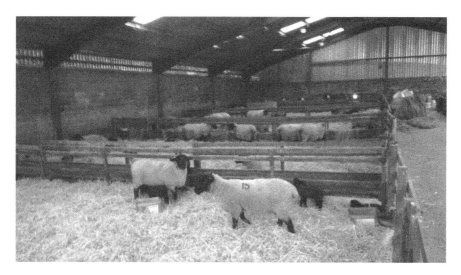

Figure 1.2 Lambing sheds need to be carefully organised to ensure ease of observation, precision nutritional management and minimal disturbance of lambing ewes.

Table 1.1 Equipment list for lambing sheep.

Suitable antiseptic solution

Obstetric lubricant

Arm length disposable gloves

Lambing ropes, snares or other aids

Clean needles and syringes

Antibiotics for treatment of mastitis or metritis

Injectable anti-inflammatory drugs

Plastic retainers or harnesses, local anaesthetic, clean obstetric tape and needles for the management of vaginal prolapse

Calcium borogluconate injection for the treatment of hypocalcaemia

Propylene glycol, or other concentrated energy supplements for the treatment of pregnancy toxaemia

Strong iodine tincture for navels and a dip cup or spray to apply

Stomach tubes, colostrum, a warming box, glucose injection, syringes and needles for the treatment of starvation and hypothermia

Kettle for hot water

Rehydration drench or formula for lambs

Clips or small syringes and needles for subconjunctival injections to correct entropion

Oral antibiotics for watery mouth prevention if needed

Injectable antibiotics for the treatment of neonatal bacteraemias if needed

Elastrator rubber rings for lambs if needed

Marker paint

Spare hurdles for making addition pens

Disinfectant for pens and floors

Sufficient clean buckets for food and water

Normal Lambing

The normal ewe gestation period is 143–147 days. Impending lambing (parturition) is signalled by udder development, accumulation of colostrum, slackening of the sacro-iliac ligaments between the tail head and the vulva and visible dropping of the abdominal contents, giving an appearance of hollowness of the sublumbar spaces on both sides of the ewe. The birth process is described as having three consecutive stages.

First stage labour is represented by cervical dilation, which takes 2–6 hours, being fastest in ewes bearing multiple lambs (multiparous ewes). Behavioural changes are often the first sign of impending lambing. The ewe will frequently separate herself from the flock or not come forward for feeding. If she does come to the trough, she may leave early. Sheep may paw at the ground and then sniff the area, while frequently lying down and then standing (Figure 1.3).

Ewes lambing outdoors often separate themselves from the flock at this stage, so it is important that corners, ditches, bushes and other such areas are checked regularly. Abdominal contractions (straining) will start, initially lasting 15–30 seconds and occurring at about 15 minute intervals. Straining becomes more frequent, until it is happening every two to three minutes, and a string of mucus may be seen at the vulva. The appearance of the water bag at the vulva indicates that the ewe is ready to give birth, although the bag may burst and go unnoticed. This process usually occurs faster in older animals which have previously given birth, and tends to be slower in ewe lambs and gimmers. Disturbance of the sheep during this process may also delay progress.

Second stage labour is represented by the passage of the lamb through the birth canal, and typically takes about one hour. The breaking of the water bag (rupture of allanto-chorion) is indicated by a rush of fluid, following which part of the

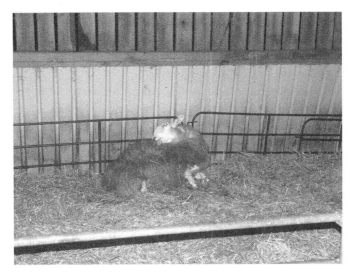

Figure 1.3 Ewes in first stage labour initially separate themselves from the main group in a preferred lambing site before abdominal contractions begin.

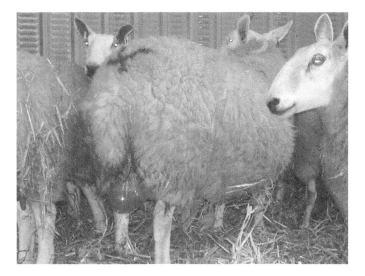

Figure 1.4 The appearance of the placenta and foetus in the birth canal indicates second stage labour.

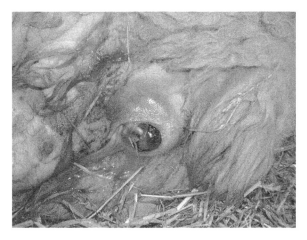

Figure 1.5 Normal unassisted delivery of a lamb in anterior presentation.

placenta (the amnion) and foetus are presented into the birth canal. Powerful reflex and voluntary contractions of abdominal muscles will occur every couple of minutes. Parts of the lamb may be seen protruding from the vulva (Figure 1.4).

Once the lamb has appeared at the vulva it is normally delivered soon afterwards (Figure 1.5). Again, disturbance of the ewe may delay this process.

Once the lamb is born, the ewe should immediately lick and clean the lamb. This process is important for stimulating the lamb and establishing the bond between mother and young, as well as drying the lamb. Ewes bearing multiple lambs may start to deliver the next within minutes, or a gap of an hour may occur. Delays greater than one hour should be considered abnormal, and the ewe should be examined.

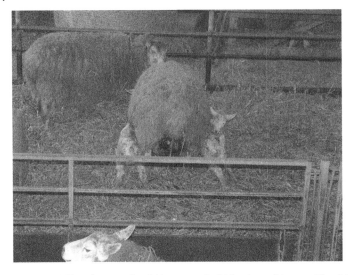

Figure 1.6 The placenta should be passed within about 3 hours of lambing.

Third stage labour is completed by expulsion of foetal membranes (placenta), which usually occurs within 2–3 hours of the end of second stage labour. The placenta may be passed at the time of lambing, or shortly afterwards (Figure 1.6). If the placenta has not been passed within three hours, the ewe should be investigated, as this could result in potentially serious infection.

The process of preparing to give birth, including dilation of the cervix and delivery of the lamb(s), takes longer in ewes lambing for the first time (primiparous), compared with animals which have given birth previously. These animals should be given sufficient undisturbed time in a quiet environment to allow the hormonal mechanisms of birth to take place. Careful, unobtrusive observation should be undertaken, to allow early detection of potential problems.

When to Intervene

Every sheep and every delivery is different, so there are no hard and fast rules for when to intervene. Intervention with lambing should only be considered when failure to do so might compromise the health of the ewe or unborn lamb. Intuitive, common sense assessment of the ewe usually gives an indication of prolonged birth stress. If the ewe lies on her side (lateral recumbency), with frequent abdominal straining and vocalisation, it may indicate that the lamb is engaged in the birth canal. Tooth grinding and, heavy breathing, involving contraction of abdominal muscles and panting, may indicate more serious concerns. Table 1.2 gives some guidelines as to when intervention and assistance should be considered.

Difficult, painful and extended lambings have serious consequences for the health and welfare of both the ewe and her lambs. The consequences of the birth of weak lambs as a result of an obstructed labour (dystocia) include an increased mortality rate, a higher incidence of neonatal infections, slower weight gain,

Table 1.2 Indications of the need to assist lambing.

The ewe has been trying to lamb for one hour without a lamb being delivered.

The interval between the water-bag breaking and expulsion of a foetus exceeds 30 minutes.

No further progress has been made 20 minutes after some of the lamb has been visible at the vulva.

Frequent powerful contractions have persisted, but no progress made in the delivery of a lamb.

The ewe appears to have started to lamb, then stopped.

The lamb's head is visible, but no forelimbs have been seen at the vulva.

Two forelimbs, but no head is seen visible at the vulva.

A foetal head and only one forelimb is seen at the vulva.

Only a tail is seen at the vulva.

A large and obviously stuck lamb is seen, sometimes with a swollen head or tongue.

Parts of two lambs are seen at the same time at the vulva.

Thirty minutes have elapsed after the birth of the first lamb, but twins or triplets are expected.

An unpleasant brown or smelly vulval discharge is noted, indicating the presence of decomposing foetuses.

Other problems, such as vaginal prolapse, have been identified.

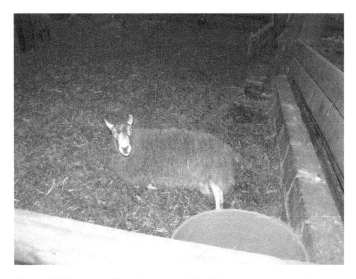

Figure 1.7 Protracted lambing or unskilled intervention can seriously compromise the health, welfare and productivity of both the ewe and her lambs.

higher medication costs and greater time spent on their care. The consequences of trauma on the ewe include reduced colostrum and milk let-down or production, poor mothering behaviour, higher medication costs, time spent on care and potentially reduced future fertility (Figure 1.7).

Prompt assistance should be given for any cases of ewes suffering dystocia. Unskilled intervention often results in swelling (oedema) and bruising of vulva, with outward evidence of vaginal bleeding on the tail and skin around the rectum and vulva (perineum). Excessive or uncontrolled force must never be used, as this endangers both mother and offspring, nor should numerous individuals attempt to lamb the same sheep. A failure to observe these measures and strict hygienic precautions often leads to womb infection (metritis).

Veterinary assistance may be appropriate when serious problems arise. It is better to seek veterinary assistance early, and minimise interference with the ewe, than to delay before having to call the vet to remove non-viable lambs from a now-debilitated animal that may subsequently die.

Factors which make veterinary assistance essential include:

i) oversized or malpresented lambs that cannot be delivered without compromising the welfare or survival of the ewe or lamb;
ii) failure of dilation of the cervix that cannot be corrected by gentle manipulation;
iii) some congenital deformities in the lamb.

If it is considered to be genuinely uneconomical or impractical to seek veterinary assistance in circumstances such as these, there must be a contingency for the immediate euthanasia of the affected ewe, to prevent further intolerable suffering. However, in calculating the economics of veterinary involvement, the cost of losing a ewe and her lambs as a result of incorrectly managed dystocia must include the lost sale value of the lambs, the replacement cost of the ewe, carcase removal or disposal charges, the cost of medicines used and staff time caring for the ewe before death.

Hygiene

To protect the ewe, the lamb and the shepherd, attention to hygiene is of paramount importance during the examination of lambing ewes and assisted lambings. Using dirty, ungloved hands to lamb a ewe can result in potentially fatal infection of the womb (metritis). Even less serious womb infections result in reduced milk production, with consequences of poor lamb growth, increased lamb losses and associated treatment costs.

Wherever possible, hands should be thoroughly washed with water and an antibacterial soap, or a dilute solution of a disinfectant. In circumstances where no anti-bacterial cleanser is available, a thorough wash with soap and hot water will often be adequate. Protective arm-length gloves must be worn whenever hand washing is impractical. It can also be helpful to wash the vulva of the ewe prior to starting the examination, to prevent surface bacteria from being carried inside. Shearing of wool from around the vulva (dagging) well before the start of lambing may be advantageous, as this reduces the risk of contamination from faecal bacteria harboured in the wool.

Clean, disposable arm-length gloves should be used to improve hygiene and to prevent the spread of disease between animals and humans (zoonotic spread). While some operators dislike the use of gloves, with practice, their use becomes quite normal. Gloves also have the advantages that they work well with lubricant and that, once soiled, they can be discarded, so the operator's hands and arms remain relatively clean and odour-free.

Lubrication

Use of obstetrical lubricant is essential when performing an assisted lambing. It eases the act of lambing, making the ewe feel more comfortable, and reduces physical trauma to the ewe, with resultant better milk production and mothering behaviour in the post-lambing period. Obstetrical lubricant is usually water-based, and mixing water with lubricant may increase its effectiveness by making the area more slippery. In circumstances where no lubricant is available, a copious lather of mild soap and water is sometimes used. However, this is a poor second choice, as even mild soap may cause irritation to the vagina.

Gentle Manipulation

All assisted deliveries should be performed gently. The lamb should be handled carefully to correct mal-presentations, guarding against tears to the uterus. Particular attention should be paid to protecting the uterine wall from tears caused by the points of the lamb's hooves when repositioning legs. Excessive traction should never be used, as this can seriously reduce lamb viability and cause maternal trauma (Figure 1.8). This is particularly true in cases where the head and legs of the foetus have not properly engaged into the ewe's pelvis.

Key points are summarised in Table 1.3.

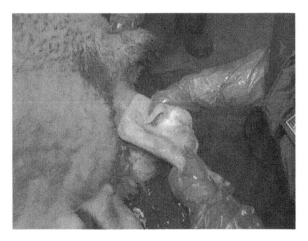

Figure 1.8 Assistance of lambing ewes requires good hygiene, lubrication and gentleness.

Table 1.3 Rules for lambing ewes.

Be vigilant	Observe ewes for signs of lambing and progress.
Be calm and quiet	Avoid disturbing ewes as much as possible.
Be prepared	Acquire all lambing supplies well before lambing, and store appropriately in an accessible box or crate.
Be clean	Wash hands, equipment and the ewe's vulva before examining or assisting with a lambing. Wear gloves.
Be gentle	Do not pull too hard. Protect the uterus from tears by fingers or the lamb's hoof.
Use plenty of lubrication	
Know your limits	Do not persevere trying to lamb a sheep beyond 5–10 minutes if you are making no progress. Know when to call for assistance.

Obstetrical Techniques

The normal position, known as the presentation, for a lamb to be born is with the nose placed upon the forelimbs with both elbows bent (Figure 1.9).

When presented with a lamb in this position, first check that there is enough space within the birth canal for the lamb to pass through. Assess the size of the lamb's hooves and head and, if necessary, place a clean, lubricated hand inside the ewe's vagina and run it around the lamb to check for any obstructions. Feel along one leg to the shoulder, across the neck and head, the other shoulder and down the other front leg, in order to ensure that all the presented parts belong to the same lamb (Figure 1.10).

Now, carefully grasping one foreleg just above the hoof, gently extend the leg to straighten the elbow. Repeat this for the other leg. Then grasp both forelimbs somewhere between the elbow and wrist (carpus), using the fingers of one hand. Run the other hand over the top of the lamb's head, so that the fingers find purchase on the bones of the skull at the back of the head. Pull the lamb backwards and downwards (away from the ewe's head and towards her back feet) in an arc of a quarter circle. The lamb should come smoothly. If the ewe is still contracting, then it is important to work with her contractions. Once delivered, clear the lamb's nose and mouth and place it so that the ewe can nurse it. Palpate the ewe's abdomen, to consider if there are other lambs still inside, and be prepared to assist these only if appropriate. Check the ewe's udder for colostrum.

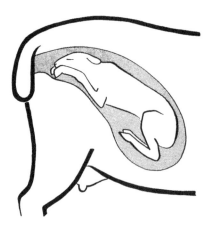

Figure 1.9 Normal presentation of a lamb or kid.

Leg Back Presentation (the nose and one leg in the birth canal)

Having determined the absence of a fore-leg in the ewe's birth canal, it is next necessary to check with a clean, lubricated hand that the head and leg presented belong to the same lamb. With a small lamb, it may be possible to retrieve the missing leg by inserting a hand along the side of the lamb's head and down to the shoulder of the absent leg. Now work the fingers down to the elbow and then gently manipulate the leg up into position, being careful to shield the hoof, to prevent tearing of the uterus. Once both feet are present, the ewe can be lambed as normal.

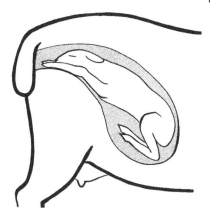

Figure 1.10 The lamb's forelegs are extended in the correct position for assisted lambing.

More commonly, there is insufficient space within the birth canal to perform this procedure with the lamb in position. In this circumstance, it is necessary to push the lamb back gently into the uterus (retropulsion), in order to locate and tweak the missing leg into position. It is advisable to place lambing ropes, as described below, on the presented parts before pushing back inside, in order to aid later retrieval.

Head Back Presentation (two legs and no head in the birth canal)

Having determined the presence of limbs, but the absence of a head in the ewe's birth canal, check that the limbs presented are both front legs by feeling the joints working up the leg, while envisaging the anatomy and nature of the joints of a lamb (Figure 1.11). To state the obvious, front legs have an elbow and hind legs a hock.

Now check that the two legs are attached to the same lamb. It can be helpful to place lambing ropes on both legs, as described below, in case the legs slip back inside.

Now run a hand over the lamb's shoulder blade, up onto its neck and along to the back of its head. Run the hand over the skull from the nearer to the further away ear, and then onto the further away side of the lamb's face. Use the fingers to bring the lamb's head round to the straight position, and then hook the fingers gently around the back of the lamb's skull and draw the head up to the pelvis.

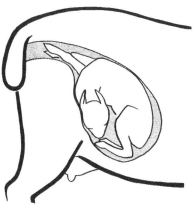

Figure 1.11 Head back presentation of a lamb or kid.

If either leg has slipped back inside the ewe's uterus, retrieve it now, while keeping the head in the correct position.

If there is room within the pelvis to allow the lamb's head to pass with a hand around it, then deliver the lamb, otherwise apply a head rope or a lambing snare, as described below, to guide the head into the pelvis while applying gentle traction to the legs to deliver the lamb.

Head Only Presentation

Having determined only the presence of a head, but no limbs, in the ewe's birth canal (Figure 1.12), it is first necessary to correctly place a head rope, as described below. Next, apply a generous amount of lubricant and with clean hands push the lamb's head back into the womb. Now retrieve the legs as described above and lamb the ewe. When the head only is presented through the birth canal, it rapidly begins to swell, making manipulation difficult and eventually causing the death of the lamb.

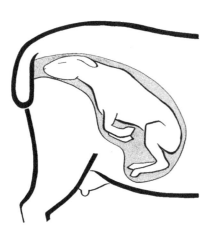

Figure 1.12 Head only presentation with bilateral shoulder flexion of a lamb or kid.

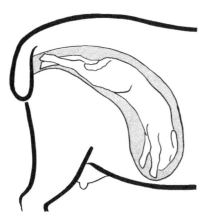

Figure 1.13 Backwards (posterior) presentation of a lamb or kid.

Backwards Presentation

Backwards presentation is identified by the presence of two back legs in the birth canal (Figure 1.13). These are confirmed as being back legs by the soles of the feet facing up towards the ewe's tail head, and the presence of the hock joints.

Feel along the inside of the legs and the tail, and identify the hindquarters in between the legs, confirming that the lamb is coming backwards, and that both legs are attached to the same lamb. Now bring the legs out to the level of the hocks, apply more lubrication and deliver the lamb, in one smooth, arc-like motion, arcing downwards (back and towards the ewe's back feet). Try not to stop during the delivery, as this can cause the lamb to inhale the birth fluids.

Beware of trying to deliver a large single lamb backwards, particularly in a terminal sire breed, as these may get stuck behind the rib cage, causing trauma or leading to inhalation of foetal fluids by the lamb.

One Back Leg Presentation

Presentation of a single back leg in the ewe's birth canal is unusual. First check that the sole of the foot points up, the leg slopes up to the hock, and that the tail and hindquarters can be felt. Usually, it is necessary to push the lamb's hindquarters away slightly, in order to make some space. Feel down the hindquarters on the side of the missing leg, feeling down that side to find the hock. Now draw the hock back slightly to bring the leg backwards. Feel down the leg to the foot and cup the foot in the hand, bringing it upwards while pushing the hock away and down. The foot should now pop around to point backwards. It is very important to cup the foot within the hand, to protect the uterine wall from the hoof – otherwise, there is a significant risk of the hoof tearing the uterine wall. Once both legs point backwards, then the ewe can be lambed as described for a posterior presentation.

Breech Presentation (tail only in the birth canal)

Breech presentation is identified by the presence of a lamb's tail, but no corresponding limbs in the birth canal (Figure 1.14). Using clean hands and generous lubrication, push the lamb's hindquarters back into the womb (retropulsion). Now retrieve both back legs, using the procedure described above, and being careful to avoid tearing. Now deliver the lamb.

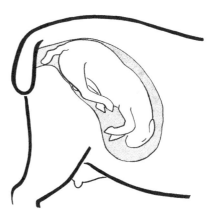

Figure 1.14 Breech, or tail only presentation of a lamb or kid.

Two Lambs Presented Together

A jumble of legs and heads in the birth canal can initially feel very confusing (Figure 1.15).

Solving the problem requires a careful and thoughtful approach. First use a clean lubricated hand to gently feel each leg, working out if it is a front or back leg, and what it is attached to. Try to visualise the problem. Having made a decision about which lamb is which, and which way round the lambs are laying, gently push one lamb back inside the womb. Now deliver the first lamb. Clear the lamb's nose and throat to stimulate it and give it to the dam. Now

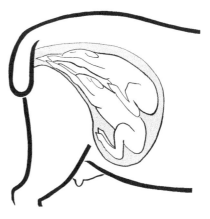

Figure 1.15 Two lambs or kids normally presented together in the birth canal.

locate the second lamb, identify the legs and head, or both back legs, and deliver the second lamb.

Correct Placement of Lambing Ropes or Snares

The traditional lambing rope is a short, soft braided rope, fitted with loops at each end. The loops are made into a noose and placed above the wrist (carpus) of the forelimbs (Figure 1.16) or ankle (tarsus) of the pelvic limbs (Figure 1.17). When used to secure the head, the noose of the rope should be placed in the lamb's mouth, then passed over the top of the skull and behind both ears (Figure 1.18).

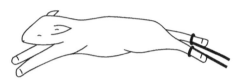

Figure 1.16 Correct placement of a lambing rope above the carpus (wrist) of a lamb.

The noose of the rope should never be placed around the lamb's neck or jaw. Ropes are best used to secure a leg or head that has to be moved to allow the lamb to be repositioned, and should never be used as a means of applying excessive traction. Plastic lambing snares can be used in a similar manner to head ropes.

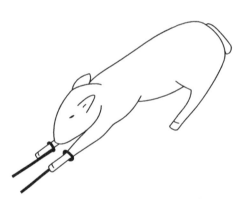

Figure 1.17 Correct placement of a lambing rope above the tarsus (ankle) of a lamb.

Ringwomb

Ringwomb is a general term used to indicate a failure of dilation of the cervix to allow the passage of the lambs into the vagina. Typically, when performing a vaginal examination of the affected sheep, the cervix is felt as a tight band constricting the birth canal, through which only 1–3 fingers can pass. The head or feet of a lamb can usually be felt beyond the cervix. Some suspected cases of ringwomb will actually be ewes in first stage labour which have been examined too early. This may particularly be the case when large groups of sheep are managed together indoors. Care should be taken to observe the sheep closely enough to avoid this situation.

Low maternal blood calcium has been implicated, but not proven, in

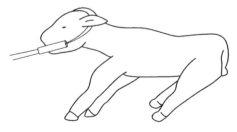

Figure 1.18 Correct placement of a lambing snare on the head of a lamb.

some cases of ringwomb. Calcium is required for muscle contraction so, in some cases, administration of injectable calcium borogluconate to the ewe may be helpful. The use of muscle relaxant drugs is rarely effective in cases of ringwomb. Gentle spreading of the cervix with the fingers is sometimes effective in dilating the cervix sufficiently to allow the delivery of the lambs, but this is impossible in ewes where the cervix will only admit a single finger. If gentle manual spreading has not dilated the cervix sufficiently to allow delivery of the lambs within 10–15 minutes, or is accompanied by bleeding, then it is unlikely that this will be effective, and veterinary attention should be sought.

Uterine Torsion

Uterine torsion is an unusual condition, characterised by straining, but failure to identify a cervical opening or passage through the vagina into the uterus. Thin spiral folds are sometimes palpable in the vaginal wall. The incidence is highest in thin ewes carrying a large single foetus. Some cases can be corrected by casting the ewe and rolling her in the perceived direction of the torsion. However, most require veterinary assistance and delivery of the lamb by Caesarean section.

Rupture of the Uterus

Excessive manual interference can cause rupture of the uterus, with subsequent shock, acute peritonitis and death of the ewe. Ewes are often anaemic and present with fast, shallow abdominal breathing, a rapid pulse and abdominal straining. Bright red arterial blood is often seen at the vulva and over the wool of the hindquarters.

Dead Lambs

Assisted delivery of dead lambs can be problematic, because the birth canal is often dry and the ewe is often sick or exhausted. If the lambs have been dead for some time, their bodies may be swollen with gas or fluid. Ewes with dead lambs inside their wombs are at a very high risk of developing serious infections. When delivering dead lambs, special attention should be paid to hygiene and lubrication. Lubricant should be generously applied, both to hand and arms, and squirted into the birth canal. Manipulation of the foetus inside the ewe should be slow and gentle, as the uterus may be prone to tearing.

In some cases of head-only presentation of lambs, where the head has passed through the birth canal, the swelling may make it impossible to push (repel) the head back into the womb to create space to retrieve the legs. The lamb is often dead by this stage, in which case it is helpful to carefully remove the head using a sharp knife. This must be done skilfully to avoid the risk of accidental damage to the ewe, and only when it is certain that the lamb is dead. The rest of the foetus can then usually be easily pushed back into the uterus, the front legs retrieved, and the ewe lambed as normal. Care should be taken to protect the birth canal from trauma caused by the stump of the severed neck.

Ewes should be treated with antibiotics for 3–5 days following the delivery of dead and decomposing lambs. An injection of non-steroidal anti-inflammatory drug (NSAID) should also be administered to the ewe. This may help to counter the action of some of the toxins she will have absorbed, and will speed her recovery by reducing pain and inflammation.

Caesarean Section

Caesarean operations (C-section) can be carried out quickly and effectively on sheep, with little impact on mothering ability or future fertility. Caesarean section can only be undertaken by a veterinary surgeon. The vet will usually be able to deliver the lambs by this route in the same state that they were in when he or she started the operation. This means that one of the most important factors affecting lamb viability is making a decision to call for veterinary assistance early on, while the lambs are still strong and viable.

Having made the decision that a caesarean might be the most appropriate option, there are several things that can be done while waiting for the vet to arrive that will maximise the chances of a successful outcome. Move the ewe to a clean, well-lit and sheltered area. A clean area will reduce contamination of the surgical site, reducing the risk of post-operative infections. Good lighting will aid the vet in performing the surgery cleanly and efficiently. Strong draughts may result in contaminants blowing into the wound, or even result in some lighter items from the vet's surgical kit blowing away.

Some vets prefer to operate on a low table-like surface, such as may be quickly constructed from straw bales or pallets, while others will prefer to operate on the ground, in which case a comfortable bed of clean straw should be provided. Most vets will prefer also to have a small table for their instruments, such as a bale or an upturned box. This will help to prevent contamination or loss of surgical instruments.

The left flank of the sheep should be clipped from two inches in front of the last rib as far as the back leg, and from the pin bones down to the belly. Wool should never be plucked.

Two spotlessly clean buckets should be filled with clean, warm water just before the vet's arrival. It is also a good idea to wash your own hands well with soap and water, to reduce contamination. The vet will need at least one person to help them by holding the sheep. When the vet is ready, lay the ewe down on its right side (left side up) and hold it down, by applying gentle pressure to the shoulder. Make sure that you are relatively comfortable, and that one or both of your hands are free. The vet will give injections of antibiotic, anti-inflammatory drugs and inject local anaesthetic, and will then prepare him/herself and the surgical site, using water, antiseptic scrub and surgical spirit. The vet is now ready to operate.

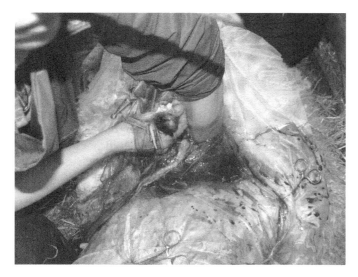

Figure 1.19 Delivery of a lamb by caesarean section. Thorough preparation and good aftercare of the ewe and lambs are critical to the success of the veterinary procedure.

The vet will cut through the skin and muscle layers and enter the abdomen, find the uterus (womb) and identify the correct site to cut. The vet will then cut into the uterus, reach inside and remove the lamb (Figure 1.19).

Frequently, the vet will pass this lamb to an assistant to revive. Once the lamb is breathing and rubbed dry, it is given to the ewe to lick, which is important to establish maternal bonding. The vet will then locate and remove any other lambs. Usually, all the lambs come out through the same incision in the uterus. Once all the lambs have been removed, the vet will suture the uterus closed, and then the body wall. Occasionally, you may be asked to assist the vet by holding things. In this case, push up your sleeves and wash your hands thoroughly. After this point, you should not touch anything at all unless specifically asked to do so.

Following surgery, the lambs should be fed colostrum, either by stomach tube or by natural sucking. The ewe and lambs should be moved to a clean, well bedded individual pen initially, with food and water for the mother. Particular attention should be paid to monitoring the subsequent health of the ewe and lambs. The dam should be injected with antibiotics for three to five days following the operation. Sometimes, stitches will need to be removed after about ten days.

Resuscitation of Newborn Lambs and Kids

Upon delivery, immediately clear any fluids from the nose, mouth and throat, using fingers, and then vigorously rub the chest using straw or a towel. If required, a piece of straw may be placed inside the nostril and wiggled to stimulate the lamb. The practice of swinging the lamb by its hind limbs underarm may be attempted, though its real effectiveness is dubious. This should be done gently and only once or twice, looking around first to avoid striking the lamb's head against an obstacle. If it is suspected that the lamb may have inhaled some birth fluids, hold its back legs up in the air so that its head hangs straight down, and gently massage the chest to encourage drainage of fluid from the lungs (the benefits of this practice are also dubious, and fluid seen coming from the lamb's mouth and nose is usually amniotic fluid from its stomach).

If the lamb still is not breathing, it may be helpful to administer a respiratory stimulant, such as one drop of doxapram under the tongue, although the benefits of this are also questionable. Lambs which have suffered significant birth stress may benefit from the administration of a low dose of a NSAID, such as flunixin or meloxicam. NSAIDs should not be administered to young goat kids, as they can cause toxicity.

Retained Placenta

Failure to pass the placenta is unusual in sheep and goats. In cases where the placenta has not been passed within 4–6 hours, antibiotic injection should be given and the lambs or kids encouraged to suck from the mother. Suckling causes the mother to produce the hormone oxytocin, which can aid the passage of the placenta.

Care of the Dam After Assisted Lambing

Special care should be taken of dams and their offspring which have had an assisted delivery (Figure 1.20).

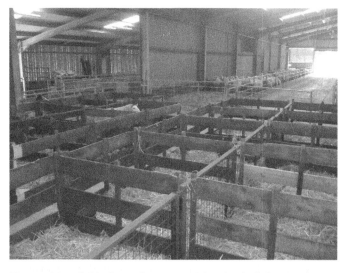

Figure 1.20 Individual pens for ewes and their lambs following the need for assisted lambing must be clean, easily accessible, well lit to allow close monitoring, draught-free and large enough to ensure that the lambs can escape being laid upon.

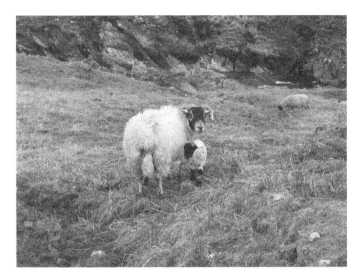

Figure 1.21 Lambing outdoors often provides a more hygienic environment than indoors. However, following assisted lambing, ewes and their lambs require shelter, easy access to food and water and routine health monitoring.

All sheep and goats that have had an assisted lambing or kidding are at increased risk of complications, and their young are more likely to suffer from starvation, hypothermia and infections. If lambing indoors, the mother and young should be moved to a clean, dry, well-bedded pen away from draughts. Water and good quality food should be freely available. Ewes and lambs should be checked frequently. If staying outside, there should be adequate shelter, water and supplementary feeding available (Figure 1.21). Outdoor ewes and lambs should be checked regularly and brought in to hospital pens if necessary.

The dam should be carefully observed for several days after an assisted lambing, for signs of a smelly discharge from the vulva, indicating metritis. Animals which have an infection, or are suffering from pain, may be less able to mother their offspring, so their lambs or kids should be carefully observed to check that they are suckling well. The dam should eat and drink, mother the lambs or kids, and should both stand and lie comfortably. Any animals where this is not the case should be examined to determine the cause of the problem, and appropriate nursing, treatment and supplementary feeding should be given.

Good nursing and regular supervision are the key to successful management of ewes and does. It is not necessary to give antibiotics to all sheep and goats which have had an assisted delivery; instead, they should be administered on a case-by-case basis, as required. Antibiotics of choice are penicillin-type drugs or oxytetracycline, and treatment should be for 3–5 days by daily injection. Care should be taken always to administer a sufficient dose of antibiotic, as under-dosing is both ineffective at treating infection and potentially causes bacteria to become resistant to the drug. Antibiotic drugs can only be prescribed by veterinary surgeons to animals under their care.

NSAIDS, such as flunixin or meloxicam, should be administered to reduce swelling in sheep and goats that have had a difficult or painful delivery, those where bruising has occurred, and those with an infection of the birth canal.

Technique for Drug Injection of Ewes

Injecting animals is not difficult, but it should always be done carefully to prevent injury. A clean needle and syringe should be used, to avoid introducing dirt or bacteria which could lead to abscess formation.

The rump (gluteal) muscles are the largest muscle mass for injection. However, the neck muscle may be preferred in fattening lambs, to avoid damaging a valuable cut of meat. It is worth noting that the sciatic nerve runs from the pelvis, across the rump and down the back of the hindlimb. It must be avoided, as damaging this nerve will result in permanent lameness. Goats tend to be bony animals, so the site for intramuscular injection should be selected carefully.

Insert the needle smoothly, draw back a little on the plunger and check that no blood has entered the hub of the needle. If blood is present, suggesting that the point is placed in a blood vessel, then withdraw the needle and try again at a different site. Injecting some drugs (for example, penicillin) into a blood vessel can be fatal. When satisfied that no blood is present, inject smoothly, then withdraw the needle and rub the injection site to disperse the drug.

Any area of loose skin can be used for subcutaneous injection. Often, the loose skin over the ribs behind the shoulder blade is a good site. Pinch up the skin to make a tent, and then insert the needle into the tent. If the syringe draws air when the plunger is pulled back, then the needle has been pushed through the other side of the skin tent and should be repositioned.

It is important not to inject large volumes of fluid that might be irritant to a single site.

Care and Management of Newborn Lambs

Lambs are most likely to survive and thrive if they are born mature, with adequate energy reserves and free from birth stress, and then receive adequate post-partum nutrition (Figure 1.22).

About 80–90% of all lamb losses are a consequence of events during the perinatal period, namely the period from birth to about one week old. Figures quoted for the incidence of perinatal lamb mortality in UK flocks range between 3–30%, although there is considerable variation within and between flocks, districts, seasons, sheep breeds, ewe age groups, farm management systems and record keeping. Perinatal lamb mortality represents a significant economic wastage, and provides an opportunity on many farms for management changes to improve the lambing percentage.

There have been several large-scale surveys of perinatal lamb mortality in a range of flock types and management systems, where dystocia linked to disproportionally high birth weights (Figure 1.23), and starvation-mismothering-exposure linked to disproportionally low birth weights (Figure 1.24) have been most often diagnosed. Dystocia may be a consequence of sire breed, the dam's pelvic conformation, maternal overfeeding, or prolonged first stage labour in multiple litters. Furthermore, dystocia injury alone may not result in lamb death, which may only occur when the lamb is subsequently subject to cold stress or

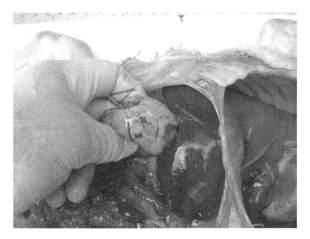

Figure 1.22 Normal, healthy, brown fat reserves over the kidneys and heart of a lamb born to a well-fed ewe.

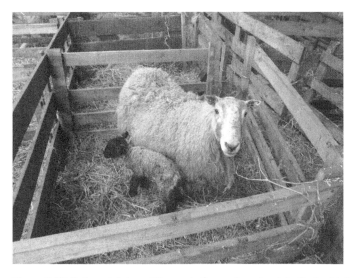

Figure 1.23 Yellow staining of the coat of a newborn lamb indicates birth stress due to dystocia, causing the meconium to be passed into the amniotic sac during parturition.

undernutrition. Likewise, starvation-mismothering-hypothermia has several causes, including dystocia.

Most newborn lamb deaths are a consequence of different combination of events occurring pre-partum, during parturition and post-partum.

Maternal Nutrition

Severe maternal under-nutrition during mid-pregnancy results in inhibited placental development, which causes poor oxygen, nutrient and electrolyte transfer to the growing foetus and, ultimately, results in poor lamb birth weights. Long

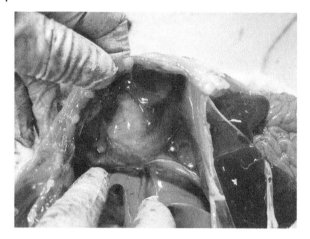

Figure 1.24 Purple colour and almost transparent brown fat over the kidneys and heart of a newborn lamb, indicating depletion of brown fat reserves and death due to starvation-mismothering-exposure.

term under-nutrition of the pregnant ewe inhibits the newborn lamb's capacity for thermoregulation, thereby increasing its susceptibility to hypothermia. Severe under-nutrition during the final six weeks of pregnancy results in the birth of lambs with low liver glycogen and brown fat energy reserves, and also in poor udder development and colostrum production for the ewe.

Overfeeding of single-bearing ewes during late pregnancy can influence the perinatal lamb mortality rate through dystocia losses of oversized lambs. Regardless of other factors, terminal sire-cross lambs with birth weights below 3.5 kg or greater than 5.5 kg suffer the highest rates of perinatal mortality.

Birth Stress

A lack of oxygen supply (anoxia) to vital centres of the central nervous system, or the compounding effect of oxygen deprivation at lambing (hypoxaemia) on pre-existing foetal low oxygen transfer (hypoxia) due to placental insufficiency, usually results in parturient foetal death. However, birth-stressed lambs do not always die during parturition. Protracted labour, compression of the umbilical cord, or mild trauma to the lamb's central nervous system during lambing can result in short-term, usually reversible, hypoxaemia of the lamb. Maintenance of body temperature, teat-searching and sucking behaviour are inhibited in surviving lambs. Furthermore, for the ewe, soft tissue trauma occurring during parturition and subsequent infection may compromise maternal behaviour, making her less likely to bond with and feed the lamb.

Post-partum Nutrition

An average 5 kg outdoor-born lamb requires about 1 litre of colostrum during its first 24 hours. Failure of the neonatal lamb to feed, or failure of the newly-lambed ewe to provide adequate colostrum, results in starvation for the lamb and poor passive immunity to disease.

Healthy lambs are born with limited energy reserves of plasma glucose and fructose, liver glycogen and brown fat. In physiologically compromised lambs, these reserves are depleted or absent. Starved lambs rapidly become hypoglycaemic and are weak, lethargic and unable to maintain body temperature.

Maternal factors responsible for lamb starvation include:

i) genotype, meaning that some individuals and certain ewe breeds demonstrate poor mothering behaviour;
ii) inexperience, for example ewe lambs and gimmers refusing to suckle their lambs;
iii) undernutrition, resulting in poor colostrum accumulation;
iv) dystocia;
v) generalised infection;
vi) mastitis;
vii) multiple births.

Lamb factors leading to starvation include:

i) genotype; for example, some terminal sire bred lambs are slower to suck than pure hill breed lambs;
ii) multiple litters, for example three lambs sharing two teats;
iii) birth stress and/or prenatal malnutrition;
iv) hypothermia, as hypothermic lambs do not feed;
v) infectious disease.

External factors responsible for lamb starvation include:

i) high stocking density of lambing ewes, resulting in mis-mothering;
ii) disturbance of lambing or newly-lambed ewes;
iii) human interference;
iv) poor pasture availability near to the lambing site;
v) exposure.

Other Causes of Perinatal Lamb Mortality

Occasionally, severe cold, wet and windy weather results in primary hypothermia, where the rate of heat loss in small lambs is so rapid that death intervenes before brown fat can be catabolised to generate heat.

Common diseases, such as non-specific bacterial septicaemias and the disease known as watery mouth, are a consequence of poor colostrum intake during the first few hours of life and poor hygiene of the lambing environment. In housed flocks, environmental contamination may become overwhelming, and infectious diseases – in particular, non-specific bacteraemias – can become important and result in significant deaths of lambs between 1–3 weeks old. In other individual flocks, navel infections, joint disease, lamb dysentery, septicaemias or diarrhoea caused by specific bacterial infections can become important, although there are usually other primary predisposing factors.

Inherited abnormalities have the potential to cause large losses, although most have been successfully controlled or eliminated in the national flock. Iodine deficiency (goitre), copper deficiency (congenital swayback) and selenium deficiency (congenital white muscle disease) have been associated with high perinatal lamb mortality rates. On some UK farms, predation by foxes or eagles can be significant, although many of the casualties are probably already compromised. Dog worrying is an increasing problem.

Management to Enhance Lamb Survival

Any management practices that ensure correct nutrition of the pregnant ewe, avoidance of dystocia, provision of energy and protective antibodies through colostrum and a strong maternal bond will enhance the perinatal lamb survival rate. However, the relative importance and practicality of such practices differ between farms.

Preparation for Lambing

Lambing is the critical time when the benefits of preparation throughout the year are realised. Lamb survival can be enhanced by planned nutritional management of the pregnant ewe.

Ewes lambing in good body condition, and which have been well fed during the final six weeks of pregnancy, suffer the lowest rates of perinatal lamb mortality. Planning is essential to ensure that ewes are mated in good body condition and correctly fed throughout pregnancy.

The maximum period of foetal growth is during the final six weeks of gestation. Nutrition during this period has a large effect on lamb birth weights, subsequent lamb viability and lamb growth rates. The mean birth weights of lambs born to adequately nourished and severely undernourished ewes are significantly different. Higher lamb mortality rates are found in triplet and twin lambs born to underfed ewes.

The use of ram harnesses or raddle (Figure 1.25) during the mating period, weighing or body condition scoring during mid-pregnancy, and ultrasound scanning for single or multiple pregnancies (Figure 1.26) are valuable management tools which can ensure that early lambing, thin or multiple-bearing ewes receive the best nutrition available.

Avoidance of Birth Stress

Lambing difficulties may arise due to presentational, positional and postural abnormalities of the foetus. Dystocia can also result from relative foetal oversize, where the foetal dimensions are normal but the ewe's pelvis is too small, and absolute foetal oversize, where the maternal pelvis is normal but the foetus is abnormally large.

Presentation and postural abnormalities are very common but are generally simple to correct, provided that they are identified early during second stage labour. When such abnormalities occur in a high proportion of the flock, a potentially excessive level of disturbance of ewes in first stage labour should be evaluated.

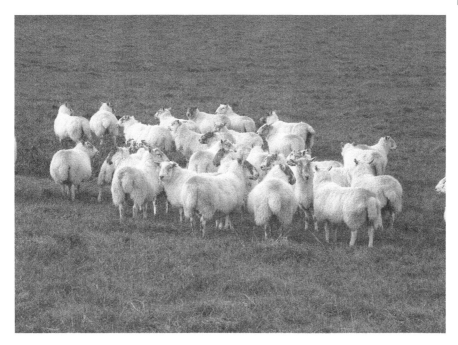

Figure 1.25 Keel or raddle marks can be used to enable precise management of ewes during late pregnancy, depending on their expected lambing date.

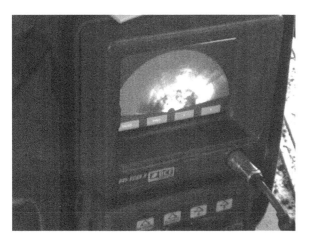

Figure 1.26 Information collected during ultrasound scanning for pregnancy can be used to enable precise management of ewes during late pregnancy, depending on foetal numbers, thereby reducing perinatal lamb mortality.

Relative foetal oversize is commonly seen in pregnant ewe lambs, because of their small pelvic diameter and relatively large foetal size. As a general rule, ewe lambs should not be mated unless they have reached about 70% of their mature adult weight, and careful consideration should be given to the choice of terminal sire. The incidence of relative foetal oversize is highest in breeds of ewe whose

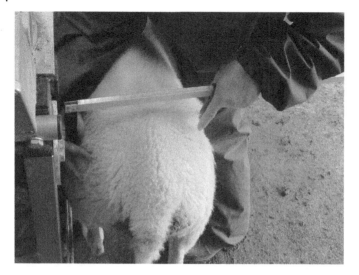

Figure 1.27 Both pelvic size and conformation (the angle at which the pelvis sits) are important with reference to dystocia.

pelvises tend to be angled forward at the base, reducing the effective area of the birth canal (Figure 1.27).

Easy Care Lambing

Easy care systems were developed in New Zealand with the original aim of reducing lamb losses to dystocia. Ease of lambing had previously been correlated to the functional area of the pelvic canal, with incompatibility in size between the maternal pelvis and the lamb at birth identified as the main cause for repeated assistance at lambing. Considerable variation had been identified within the national Romney flock, suggesting that ease of lambing might be a heritable trait. Lamb birth weight, the size and shape of the lamb's head and shoulders and limb bone thickness had also been identified as important risk factors.

Selection for ease of lambing was highly successful. However, early observations showed a disproportionally high incidence of social stress and mismothering at high stocking densities. Ewes needed to be spread out about a month before lambing commenced, so that they had time to settle down and find the warm, sheltered and dry areas. There was a need for careful pasture management to ensure pasture availability for set stocking through to the end of lambing. So long as there was sufficient pasture, ewes tended to remain at the lambing site until the lambs were strong enough to move further afield but, if pasture availability was limited, ewes tended to abandon the lambing site to look for food elsewhere, resulting in lamb losses. Human intervention of any kind invariably resulted in ewes being displaced from their lambing site and subsequent lamb losses.

Easy care lambing has been an important innovation in New Zealand sheep farming, but would be inappropriate for systems involving crossbred sheep where lambing ewes have to be disturbed to allow for supplementary feeding. Nevertheless, various measures can be taken to reduce levels of dystocia and interference with lambing ewes based on the principles of easy care lambing. Technologies such as the use of ultrasound scanning data, recording of raddle marks and blood sampling pregnant ewes to determine the adequacy of protein and energy nutrition can be used to enable more efficient pasture management at lambing and reduce the disturbance of lambing ewes.

Careful selection of lambing fields is important, and a high standard of flock health care is required to eliminate the need to disturb the whole lambing flock while treating individual sick or lame animals. Replacement ewes should be selected on the basis of external pelvic conformation, in preference to fashionable breed characteristics. Ewes which require assistance or show signs of poor mothering ability should be permanently marked and culled after weaning. Terminal sires should be selected for small heads, fine bones and narrow shoulders. Systems should be adapted to allow careful shepherding to minimise the disturbance of lambing ewes.

Adequate Lamb Nutrition

Any management practice aimed at ensuring adequate nutrition of the pregnant ewe and the prevention of dystocia will also, in turn, be beneficial to early lamb nutrition and survival. Such practices will help to ensure the birth of vigorous lambs, adequate colostrum accumulation in the ewe, the prevention of pregnancy toxaemia and mastitis and non-disturbance of the newly-lambed ewe. Additional skilled labour employed for the supervision of lambing should also be available, to ensure that lambs are correctly mothered, to supplement the nutrition of small or weak lambs, and to treat hypothermic or diseased lambs.

When provided with adequate neonatal care, even lambs suffering from mild birth stress or pre-partum undernutrition can survive. The provision of adequate shelter in lambing paddocks is an essential component of such care on all farms. The positioning of supplementary wind breaks, such as straw bales or tin sheets, should be carefully planned around the ewes' preferred lambing sites. On extensively managed hill properties, provision of shelter is paramount, because it may be the only possible method of improving conditions (Figure 1.28).

Lamb Fostering

Most ewes are unable economically to rear triplets, but most can support twins. The benefits of fostering lambs are, therefore, obvious. Several fostering methods have been described. Generally, the most successful method is to smear the orphan lamb with the foster ewe's lambing fluids immediately after the delivery of the foster ewe's lamb. It is important that the orphan lamb and the ewe's own lamb are well matched for size and that the orphan lamb is not too old. Use of ultrasound scanning results can facilitate immediate fostering of orphan lambs onto single-bearing ewes.

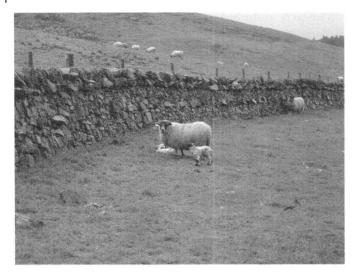

Figure 1.28 Provision of shelter may be the most pragmatic means available to improve lamb survival in extensively managed production systems.

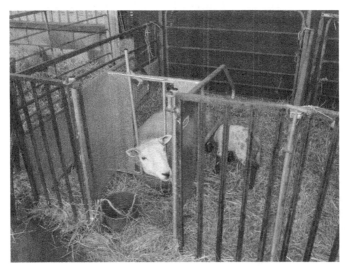

Figure 1.29 Use of 'lamb adopter' crates requires an extremely skilful level of care, to ensure adequate welfare of the ewe and lambs. Close monitoring is required after the ewe has been released.

The use of lamb adopter crates, or confinement of the ewe and lamb in a pen with the ewe tied so that she cannot injure the lambs, require skilful management to protect the welfare of the ewe and lambs (Figure 1.29). Attaching the skin of the foster ewe's own dead lamb onto the orphan lamb is sometimes successful (Figure 1.30). Alternatively, stockingette tubing cut to fit around the ewe's own lamb for a few hours, to absorb its smell and then transfer it to the fostered lamb is sometimes successful.

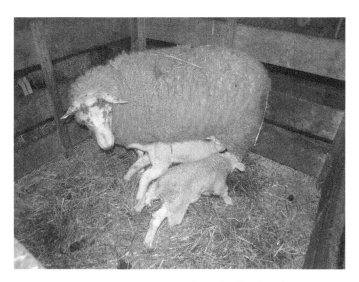

Figure 1.30 Fostering by skinning the dam's dead lamb and placing it over the surrogate lamb is not always successful. (The dead lamb is skinned by first incising the skin around each hock, and then making an incision extending from the inner aspect of one hock to that of the other. The skin is then forced away from the hindquarters, and is pulled forwards and inside-out over the body of the lamb. Incisions are then made around the elbows and neck, allowing the skin to be removed. The skin can then be turned the correct way round and fitted over the neck and forelimbs of the surrogate lamb, as shown.)

Careful monitoring is required after releasing the foster ewe and lambs. Orphan lambs often appear to follow the foster ewe at first, but are later found starving and hypothermic or dead.

Artificial Rearing

In most flocks, there will be spare lambs that cannot be fostered, and these will need to be reared artificially. Artificial rearing can be successfully achieved if the lambs are correctly and hygienically fed and kept in an appropriately pre-planned warm, clean and dry environment.

The spare lamb should ideally be left with its mother for the first 24 hours of life, supplementing colostrum for the whole litter during this period. Newborn lambs should be fed 50 ml/kg of ewe colostrum or a colostrum substitute within the first four hours of life if the ewe is sick, has rejected the lamb, or has died. The lamb should then be transferred to a warm, dry and clean environment. About 50 ml/kg of milk replacer should be fed three or four times daily, using a bottle and an appropriate teat.

Whenever possible, it is desirable to feed lambs in a natural position, as close to that of nursing from their mother, rather than restraining the lamb in an unnatural position. When first training lambs to feed from a bottle, it is helpful to have something solid behind to prevent them from reversing, while restraining them with a hand placed under the chin. Fingers should never be placed inside the lamb's mouth (Figure 1.31).

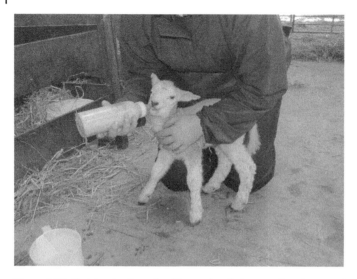

Figure 1.31 Training lambs to feed from a bottle is rewarding, but requires patience.

The lamb should be transferred to an artificial rearing pen at about three days old, provided that it is strong, sucking well and showing no signs of disease. Sick or weak lambs should never be introduced to the rearing pen. All lambs, irrespective of source or age, which are destined for artificial rearing should undergo a 48-hour quarantine period before being introduced to the communal artificial rearing pen. Lambs should be reared in small groups of up to about ten in clean, dry and draught-free pens, free from dangerous obstructions (Figure 1.32).

When using automatic milk feeders, it is sometimes necessary to increase the group size, but this increases the risk of disease spread and bullying. During the training period the rearing pen should be restricted in size but, once all the lambs are sucking well, they should be given as much space as possible, along with distractions such as footballs or straw bales to encourage playing behaviour (Figure 1.33).

If possible, feeding equipment should be cleaned daily, to prevent a build-up of faeces, urine and stale spilled milk in one area. If this is not possible, for example where static automatic feeders are used, the area around the feeder must be kept scrupulously clean and dry (Figure 1.34). In covered yards with open sides, provide straw bales arranged to form a cross, which can be used to provide shelter from draughts from all directions. These should be moved regularly to avoid build-up and concentration of pathogens. Infrared heat lamps should be avoided, because they encourage the lambs to huddle in one spot on badly soiled bedding.

Once in the rearing pens, lambs can be fed about 1–1.25 litres of replacer twice daily, although individual requirements vary greatly. Unless using automatic feeding machines that offer milk on demand, it is preferable to introduce lambs to cold milk replacer as soon as possible. Cold milk does not sour as quickly as warm milk, and lambs feed less greedily. Bottles, buckets, teats and valves should all be kept scrupulously clean and sterilised each day, using a suitable hypochlorite or detergent solution. It is important to use a good quality ewe milk replacer. These are

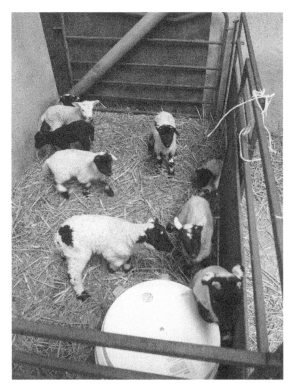

Figure 1.32 A small group of young lambs being artificially reared using a bucket-and-teat setup.

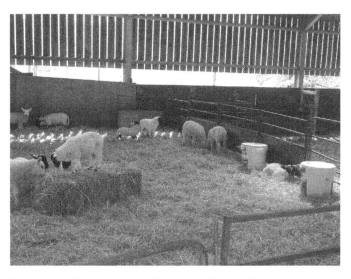

Figure 1.33 A large group of older, artificially reared lambs, provided with sufficient space and distractions to allow individuals to display natural behaviour patterns.

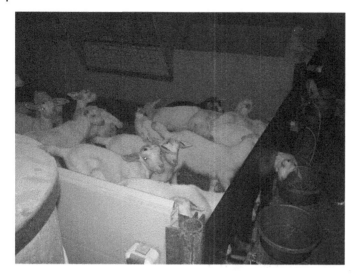

Figure 1.34 Maintaining strict hygienic conditions in the area around automatic milk replacer feeding machines is essential.

usually made up by mixing 200 g of milk powder with water to produce one litre of milk. The measure used to dispense the powder must be checked, to ensure that it gives the correct amount. If too little powder is used, the lambs may starve while, if too much is used, the lambs may scour and become dehydrated.

Lamb milk replacers have a higher fat content than calf milk replacers or cow's milk, which are generally unsuitable. Good quality hay and fresh creep feed should be made available from about one week old, to promote early rumen development. Clean, fresh water must always be available and presented in a manner such that the lambs can drink, but not drown.

If the cost of milk replacer were not a consideration, a recommendation could be made to wean all lambs from four weeks old once they reach 15 kg bodyweight. However, many artificially reared lambs will not meet this target, so a balance must be struck between the cost of milk replacer and performance of the lamb, without compromising its health and welfare.

Care must be taken not to wean lambs too early, otherwise a serious check in growth and intestinal problems will result. Lambs should not be weaned before 30 days of age or at a body weight of less than 10 kg, although common sense and experience must be applied in the application of these guidelines. Lambs must be taking solid food before weaning. Weaning of artificially reared lambs should be undertaken abruptly, otherwise strong lambs that are ready for weaning will continue to get milk while weaker lambs will not.

The relatively close confinement of lambs in an artificial rearing system inevitably increases the risk of infectious diseases. The incidence of these problems can be reduced by following the practices outlined above. Milk replacer-fed lambs are sometimes found dead, with grossly distended abdomens, about one hour after feeding. The problem is associated with overfilling of the abomasum and rapid proliferation of gas-producing organisms. The incidence of abomasal bloat is highest when lambs are fed infrequently, using warm milk replacer, encouraging greedy feeding behaviour. The problem is prevented by feeding lambs regularly with measured amounts of cold milk-replacer.

Risk of Zoonotic Diseases

Feeding pet lambs raises challenges concerning the zoonotic transmission of pathogens, such as Gram-negative toxin-producing bacteria, coccidian parasites and viruses (Figure 1.35). Distressing high-profile reports of diseases in children due to verotoxigenic *Escherichia coli*, cryptosporidiosis and orf heighten awareness of the need for basic hygienic measures, such as hand washing and avoidance of oral contact with contaminated objects, as well as the importance of controlling zoonotic diseases in general.

Alternatives to Fresh Colostrum

1) Ewes frequently have more colostrum than is immediately required by their own lambs. Excess colostrum can be milked, batched and stored or frozen in suitable small quantities. Care is needed not to overheat frozen colostrum during the thawing process.
2) Cow colostrum, procured in advance of the lambing season and frozen in small containers, is a useful alternative to ewe colostrum. Cow colostrum contains approximately 20% less energy per ml than ewes' colostrum, so correspondingly larger volumes are required. It contains some useful antibodies, but may not protect against specific pathogens found in individual flocks. Clostridial antigens can be boosted by prior immunisation of the cow with an ovine clostridial

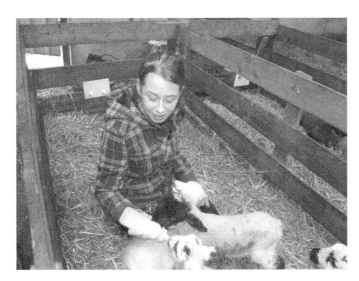

Figure 1.35 There is a strong and important bond between young children and pet or orphan lambs. However, strict hygienic precautions such as hand washing must be taken, regardless of the hygienic conditions on the farm.

vaccine. Rarely, cow colostrum contains antibodies against antigens on the lamb's red blood cells, causing severe and usually fatal anaemia when the lamb is between 10–20 days old. Pooling of colostrum from several cows will dilute the effect of any anti-sheep red blood cell antibodies present.

3) Most proprietary powdered colostrum substitutes for lambs are derived from cow colostrum, tested for anaemia-producing antibodies. Some are derived from ewe colostrum and are, therefore, superior. Powdered colostrum is convenient, although cost precludes its widespread use.

Lamb Castration

Castration is a mutilation, and should only be performed when it is necessary to do so – for example, to avoid unwanted pregnancies or to avoid the development of male secondary characteristics in lambs or kids that may be kept for longer than about six months, when they might become sexually mature.

Rubber rings are a simple and effective means of castration. Good application technique is important to prevent unnecessary injury to the lamb and potentially costly castration failures (Figure 1.36). If rubber rings are used, they must, by law, be applied within the first week of life. Most shepherds apply rings between 24 and 72 hours after birth. Application of rubber rings before 24 hours is not recommended, as this may interfere with the ingestion of colostrum and the formation of the maternal bond.

It is first necessary to check that both testicles have descended into the scrotum, and that the lamb does not have a hernia. A hernia can be felt as a soft mass of intestines within the scrotum. The procedure may be easily carried out in a seated position. The rubber ring is placed on the prongs of the applicator prior to starting. The lamb is restrained between the knees with its head up and the body extended and relaxed. The scrotum should not be touched, as this will cause the lamb to retract his testicles. Using the applicator so that the prongs point towards the lamb's body, the ring is passed over the scrotum and both testicles. The prongs are pushed slightly into the abdomen and the ring is closed (Figure 1.37). The applicator should not be withdrawn at this stage.

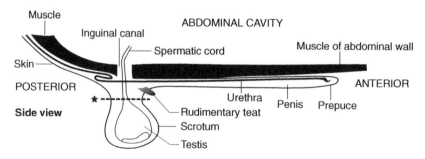

Figure 1.36 Diagram showing the male lamb scrotal anatomy, along with the correct position for placing a rubber ring.

Next, a check should be made to ensure that both testicles are trapped within the scrotum beyond the ring and that both nipples are still above the ring on the lamb's belly and have not been drawn into the ring. Should there be any problem, it is much more easily dealt with now than after the removal of the applicator. When happy that the ring is correctly located, it can be rolled off the applicator.

It is normal for lambs to show signs of pain, including lying and kicking, for a few hours after application of rubber rings. They should be checked regularly to ensure that the signs of discomfort subside, and that they are correctly mothered up. Inclusion of excessive belly skin within the ring can result in significant wounds around the area. Should these be present, they should be cleaned with water and mild disinfectant or salty water and the lamb should be given antibiotic treatment.

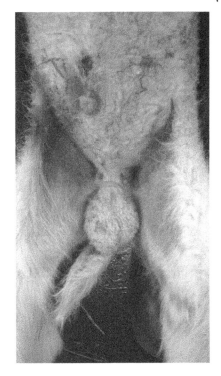

Figure 1.37 Lamb castration by correct placement of a rubber ring.

Bloodless castration is sometimes performed using precisely engineered surgical instruments, such as the Burdizzo emasculator or Ritchey Nipper. These instruments must be well maintained and handled with care to avid misalignment of the jaws, which can, in turn, result in castration failure and/or unnecessary pain or injury. These methods work on the principle that when the jaws are closed over the neck of the scrotum, the blood vessels in the spermatic cord are crushed and the scrotal contents deprived of their blood supply. The scrotum and its contents eventually shrivel and die. The scrotal skin remains intact, preventing the entry of infection.

With the lamb securely restrained, the device must be applied at two points approximately 1 cm apart, one on each side of the neck of the scrotum, along the spermatic cord (Figure 1.38). To avoid damaging the penis or urethra, the jaws must be applied well below the body wall and well above the testes. The jaws must never be placed across the whole width of the scrotal neck in a single crush. Doing this blocks the blood supply to the entire scrotum and causes pain.

As with rubber ring castration, bloodless castration requires a high level of skill and care to avoid causing unnecessary suffering. Lambs should be checked afterwards for mismothering and signs of excessive pain or swelling of the scrotal tissue. Poor technique may also lead to lambs not being properly castrated, and they should be checked again after several weeks to make sure that the procedure has been effective. Bloodless castrators must never be used for any other purpose, such as tail docking.

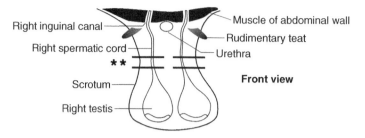

Right inguinal canal

Right spermatic cord

** **

Scrotum

Right testis

Muscle of abdominal wall

Rudimentary teat

Urethra

Front view

Figure 1.38 Diagram showing the male lamb scrotal anatomy, along with the correct positions for bloodless castration. Bloodless castration equipment should never be placed across the entire width of the scrotal neck.

While not mandatory in young lambs, veterinary advice should be sought concerning the use of local anaesthesia and/or appropriate techniques.

Application of Rubber Rings for Tail Docking

Tail docking may reduce soiling of the fleece, which may reduce incidences of flystrike. However, the procedure is a mutilation, and the benefits are contentious. Tail docking should only be undertaken where it can be justified as being beneficial to animal health and welfare.

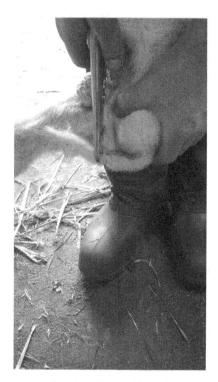

Figure 1.39 Use of a rubber ring for tail docking, showing the correct use of the applicator and placement of the ring.

Rubber rings may be used in a similar manner for tail docking of lambs, usually at the same time. Rings must be applied before seven days of age, but application before 24 hours old is not recommended.

The tail of a male fattening lamb should be long enough to cover the anus plus 2.5 cm. For a female lamb, the tail should be longer, such that it covers the vulva plus 4–6 cm. Sheep with excessively short tails may be at increased risk of flystrike and rectal prolapse.

The lamb is held in a similar manner to tail docking. The lamb's body is extended, and one leg is drawn up towards the abdomen to allow easier access to the tail. The ring is placed and its position checked before the applicator is removed (Figure 1.39). Tails have tendency to finish up shorter than expected so, if in any doubt, allow more tail at this stage.

2

Specific Causes of Lamb and Kid Mortality

Hypothermia (low body temperature)

Lamb losses to hypothermia are highest outdoors in wet, cold and windy environments but can also occur indoors, in particular in lambs that are compromised due to dystocia. Small lambs with wet birth coats are most susceptible to heat loss from exposure, while larger lambs become hypothermic, due to a combination of heat loss and starvation, sometimes secondary to infectious diseases.

In the absence of infectious abortion, lambs born to well-fed ewes generally have adequate birth weights and energy reserves, in the form of brown fat around the heart and kidneys and carbohydrates in muscle and liver tissue. These enable them to maintain body temperature for several hours after birth. The period of maintenance of body temperature is dependent on:

  i) the lamb's colostrum intake;
 ii) the ewe's mothering ability;
iii) the rate of chilling from the environment.

Once these energy reserves have been depleted, lambs rapidly become hypothermic unless they can receive sufficient colostrum and shelter to ensure that their rate of heat production exceeds their rate of heat loss.

The normal rectal temperature of newborn lambs, exhibiting normal sucking behaviour is between 39–40 °C. Moderately hypothermic lambs with rectal temperatures between 37 °C and 39 °C are weak, but are still capable of following their dam and feeding (Figure 2.1). Severely hypothermic lambs, with rectal temperatures below 37 °C, stand with an arched back, have hollow flanks and a lowered head, sometimes sheltering close to the ewe's udder and giving an impression of feeding, but are unable to suck. In the absence of human intervention, these lambs become comatose and die.

The appropriate management of hypothermic lambs depends both on their rectal temperature and on their age. Where the rectal temperature of the lamb indicates moderate hypothermia, it is usually sufficient to dry the lamb thoroughly, ensure that it takes a colostrum feed and then return it to the ewe. The ewe should be checked to identify possible predisposing causes, such as mastitis,

Practical Lambing and Lamb Care – A Veterinary Guide, Fourth Edition.
Neil Sargison, James Patrick Crilly and Andrew Hopker.
© 2018 John Wiley & Sons Ltd. Published 2018 by John Wiley & Sons Ltd.

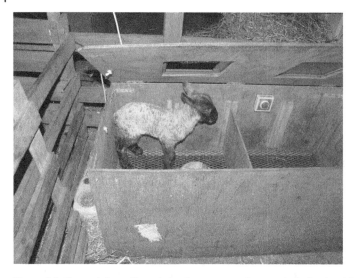

Figure 2.1 Severely hypothermic lambs may stay close to their dam's udder, but are unable to suck and will die unless they are identified and treated. The lamb has been transferred to a warming box following treatment.

systemic illness or poor mothering behaviour, and the lamb should be closely monitored.

Where the rectal temperature of the lamb indicates severe hypothermia, and the lamb is known to be less than five hours old, it can be assumed that its energy reserves have not yet been depleted. The lamb should be thoroughly dried, then warmed until its rectal temperature exceeds 37 °C, before giving a colostrum feed at a rate of 50 ml/kg. Feeding the lamb before warming may result in regurgitation or overspill of the colostrum into the lamb's lungs. The lamb should then be warmed until its rectal temperature is 39–40 °C before returning it to the ewe. Again, the ewe should be checked and the lamb should be closely monitored.

Where the rectal temperature of the lamb indicates severe hypothermia and the lamb is, or may be, more than five hours old, it should be assumed that its energy reserves are depleted. Warming the lamb will induce fitting behaviour and death, as the metabolic requirements of the brain for energy cannot be met. The lamb should first be given an intraperitoneal injection of 20% glucose at a rate of 10 ml/kg, as described below. It should then be thoroughly dried and warmed until its rectal temperature exceeds 37 °C, before giving a colostrum feed at a rate of 50 ml/kg. The lamb should then be warmed until its rectal temperature is 39–40 °C, then returned to the ewe. The ewe should be checked and the lamb should be closely monitored (Figure 2.2).

Lambing buildings should be draught-free. Shelter from wind and rain prevailing from all directions should be available, or created in outdoor lambing fields.

Prevention of hypothermia relies on:

i) ensuring that pregnant ewes are adequately fed;
ii) avoiding dystocia problems;

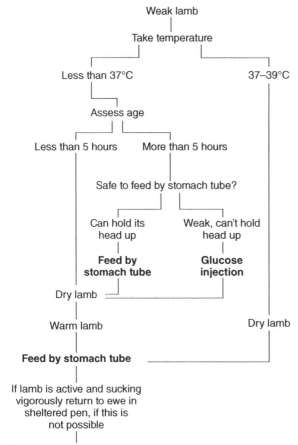

Figure 2.2 Flow chart for the correct treatment of moderately (rectal temperature between 39–37 °C) and extremely hypothermic (rectal temperature less than 37 °C).

iii) providing sufficient skilled labour to ensure that newborn lambs feed within the first few hours of life;
iv) prevention of neonatal infectious diseases;
 v) provision of adequate shelter.

Intraperitoneal Glucose Injection

The 20% glucose solution used for intraperitoneal injection should be warmed to body temperature. A practical approach is to add an equal volume of boiled water to a 40% glucose solution, then allow it to cool to about 39 °C. The lamb is then held by its pelvic limbs, facing away from the operator. A 2 cm² area is cleaned and dabbed with disinfectant, about 2 cm to the side of and 2 cm below the navel. A 19-gauge one-inch needle is then inserted into the peritoneal cavity, directed towards the tail head (Figure 2.3).

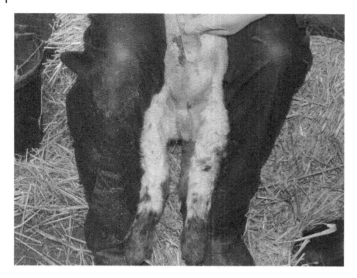

Figure 2.3 Intraperitoneal glucose injection.

Using this method, the peritoneal organs fall away from the point of the needle and are not punctured. The warmed glucose solution is then injected slowly. It is normal for the lamb to urinate as the warmed fluid is injected. Glucose injections should never be given subcutaneously as this may cause severe irritation, sometimes leading to sloughing of the skin. In fact, glucose administered under the skin is poorly absorbed by hypothermic animals.

Warming boxes which provide a thermostatically regulated all-round heat source are preferable to heat lamps or hot water bottles, which only warm one surface of the lamb (Figure 2.4).

The warming box works on the principle that the lamb is laid on a rack or mesh shelf inside a box, and warm air provided from a fan heater below can circulate around the lamb's body. The temperature inside the box must be monitored, and can be controlled by opening or closing the lid of the box to ensure that the lamb does not overheat (Figure 2.5).

It is possible to build a makeshift warmer box using straw bales (Figure 2.6). This can have the benefit of being able to be rebuilt regularly, and recycled to reduce the build-up of disease contamination. Great care must be taken to monitor and regulate the temperature inside these arrangements. Any fire risk must also be accounted for.

Feeding Lambs by Stomach Tube

Lambs which are unable to suck from a teat should be fed using a stomach tube and feeder. Only proprietary lamb stomach tubes should be used, as these are designed to be placed into the stomach easily and correctly while avoiding injury. The tube should first be placed in warm water to soften the plastic. This can be done while the colostrum, milk, or glucose and electrolyte solution to be fed is

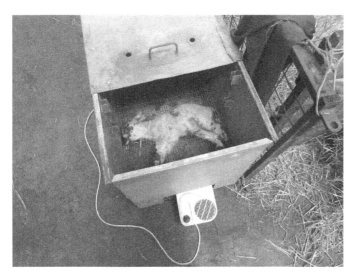

Figure 2.4 A commercially manufactured lamb warming box, providing all-round heat and control of the temperature inside.

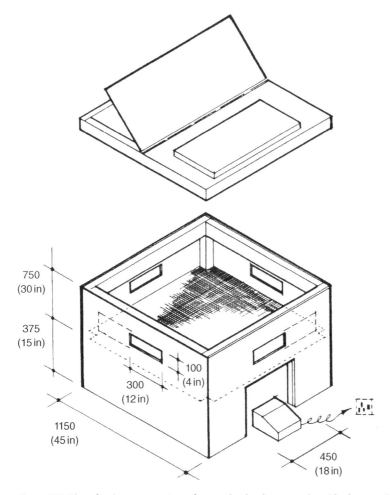

750
(30 in)

375
(15 in)

100
(4 in)

300
(12 in)

1150
(45 in)

450
(18 in)

Figure 2.5 Plans for the construction of a wooden lamb warmer box. The box can be partitioned to allow several lambs to be warmed without risking cross contamination and spread of disease.

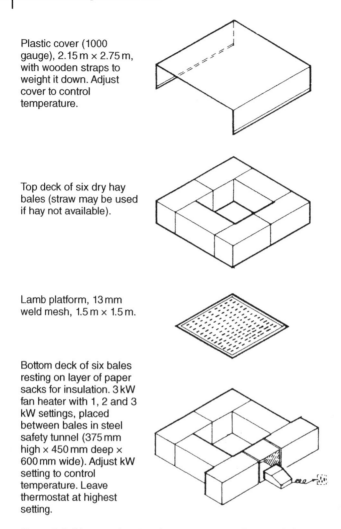

Plastic cover (1000 gauge), 2.15 m × 2.75 m, with wooden straps to weight it down. Adjust cover to control temperature.

Top deck of six dry hay bales (straw may be used if hay not available).

Lamb platform, 13 mm weld mesh, 1.5 m × 1.5 m.

Bottom deck of six bales resting on layer of paper sacks for insulation. 3 kW fan heater with 1, 2 and 3 kW settings, placed between bales in steel safety tunnel (375 mm high × 450 mm deep × 600 mm wide). Adjust kW setting to control temperature. Leave thermostat at highest setting.

Figure 2.6 Diagram showing the construction of a straw bale warmer.

being prepared to the correct temperature. The lamb should be gently, but firmly, restrained between the knees of the operator, with its head up and body straight. A hand is placed under the lamb's chin and the mouth is gently opened just far enough to insert the tube over the tongue. The empty tube then is advanced as the lamb swallows (Figure 2.7).

The tube is held close to the mouth, to prevent it flexing as it is advanced. The lamb's swallowing reflex indicates that the tube is correctly placed, while attempts to cough or gag suggest that it is not. The feeder is filled only when the tube is placed, and is then allowed to flow freely and drain completely before withdrawing (Figure 2.8). The tube should be withdrawn quickly and smoothly to avoid any remaining fluid trickling into the larynx and lungs. The apparatus should be thoroughly cleaned between uses.

Disposable latex or nitrile gloves should be worn when handling the mouths of young lambs to minimise the spread of zoonotic infections such as orf.

Watery Mouth

Watery mouth is a common disease of one- to three-day-old lambs seen under all management systems. The clinical signs begin with depression, loss of appetite (anorexia) and, frequently, hypothermia, and rapidly progress to recumbency and collapse. The mouth is cold and the angles of the lips and the lower are jaw wet due to drooling of saliva (Figure 2.9).

Lambs are frequently dehydrated, with abdominal distension. The rectal temperature may be normal, but the extremities are often cold. Mucous membranes of the conjunctivae of the eyes are congested, and scleral blood vessels in the eyes are dilated. Abdominal palpation is clearly resented, and there are usually insufficient faeces in the rectum to stain a thermometer.

Losses can be particularly high in indoor flocks during the second and subsequent weeks of lambing. Triplets are three times more likely to be affected than are single and twin lambs. The response to treatment with the anti-endotoxic NSAID drug flunixin, fluids and systemic antibiotics is poor, so therefore the emphasis must be on prevention.

Watery mouth follows reduced or delayed colostrum intake. The pH of the lamb's stomach (abomasum) before taking its first feed of colostrum is neutral. This is a physiological mechanism which enables antibodies in the colostrum to pass undamaged to their site of absorption in the small intestine. However, the neutral pH also allows passage through the stomach, and rapid multiplication of faecal *Escherichia coli* bacteria. These bacteria are acquired soon after birth, during teat searching, from the ewe's contaminated fleece and udder. Toxins are released on the death of the

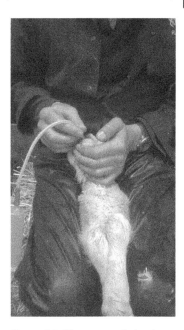

Figure 2.7 Placement of a lamb stomach tube for supplementary colostrum feeding.

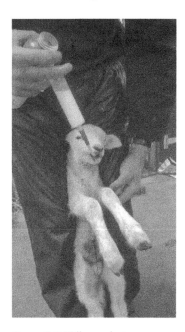

Figure 2.8 Milk or colostrum should flow naturally through the stomach tube apparatus. A maximum of 50 ml per kg lamb weight can be fed at one time.

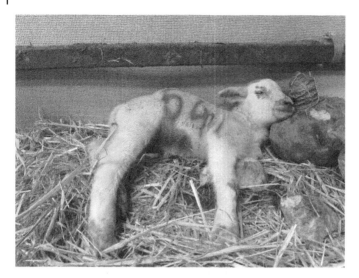

Figure 2.9 Distended abomasum and saliva under the chin in a typical clinical presentation of watery mouth in a lamb.

bacteria from their cell walls (endotoxins), and these are responsible for the clinical signs of watery mouth (generalised endotoxaemia).

Prevention of watery mouth depends on correct nutrition of the pregnant ewe and management of dystocia, as well as on the maintenance of a clean lambing environment. Adequate supervision is needed to ensure that all lambs feed or receive 50 ml/kg of colostrum or colostrum substitutes by stomach tube within their first hour of life.

On many farms, the preventive (prophylactic) oral administration of specific antibiotic drugs (usually aminoglycoside antibiotics such as apramycin, neomycin and spectinomycin, or amoxicillin), to all lambs within 15 minutes of birth, is practised (Figure 2.10). Good results are attributed to suppression of *E. coli* multiplication in the intestinal lumen. However, this strategy is not a substitute for good husbandry and management, and should be avoided or minimised to reduce the risk of selection for antimicrobial drug resistance.

Lamb Dysentery

Lamb dysentery is a sudden onset fatal clostridial disease of young lambs (Figure 2.11). Affected lambs are usually less than two weeks old and, most commonly, are one to three days old. Most cases occur in stronger single lambs that had previously been consuming the largest quantities of milk. Serious outbreaks of lamb dysentery are sometimes seen during cold and wet springs, when lambing ewes are confined to small sheltered areas and conditions become unhygienic. In extreme cases, losses due to lamb dysentery of between 20–30% have been reported.

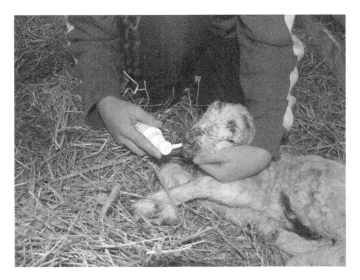

Figure 2.10 Prophylactic oral administration of antibiotic drugs can be helpful in reducing the incidence of watery mouth. However, this is not an alternative for good hygiene and colostrum management, and it may prove to be irresponsible in selecting for antimicrobial resistance.

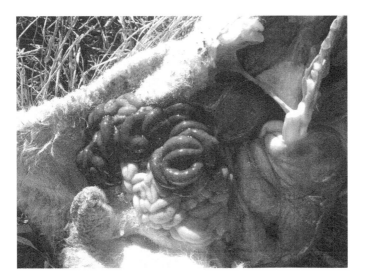

Figure 2.11 Lamb dysentery usually presents as sudden death. The diagnosis is based on post-mortem findings of localised areas of dark, red-coloured intestinal distension, with blood-stained peritoneal fluid.

Effective prevention of lamb dysentery is achieved through vaccination of ewes, using a multi-component vaccine containing toxoids of *Clostridium perfringens* type B in an adjuvant. Vaccination of ewes protects their newborn lambs through colostral transfer of passive immunity.

Enterotoxigenic *Escherichia coli*

Enterotoxigenic *E. coli* attach to the small intestinal mucosa during the first 24 hours of life, then produce a toxin that causes severe watery, brown-coloured diarrhoea. Disease outbreaks are uncommon, but can cause significant losses. Most affected lambs die unless prompt fluid therapy is administered.

Control and prevention of enterotoxigenic *E. coli* depends on strict hygiene, ensuring adequate early colostrum intake and immediate isolation of sick lambs.

Cryptosporidiosis

The single-cell (protozoan) intra-cellular (coccidian) parasite *Cryptosporidium parvum* is not species-specific and hence, potentially, can infect humans (zoonotic). *C. parvum* infection damages the cells lining the small intestine, reducing its capacity to absorb nutrients (malabsorption) or exchange nutrients (by causing villous atrophy), leading to diarrhoea. *C. parvum* alone seldom causes severe disease in lambs. However, if environmental contamination with the infective stages of the parasite (oocysts) is high, or if the lambs are otherwise compromised or stressed, the parasite may cause acute onset, pale green-coloured, watery and occasionally blood-stained diarrhoea in lambs between 2–20 days old. Large numbers of lambs may be affected and, if they are not promptly treated, mortalities can occur (Figure 2.12). Cryptosporidiosis is a potentially serious zoonosis.

Anti-coccidial agents used for the treatment and prevention of coccidiosis in older lambs are ineffective for the control or treatment of cryptosporidiosis, so

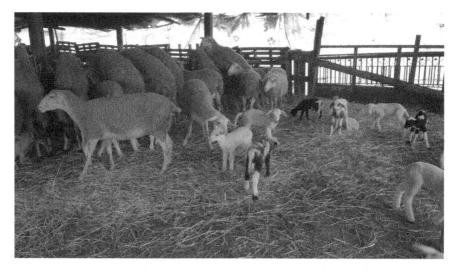

Figure 2.12 Keeping young lambs in large groups in cold and damp pens increases the risk of cryptosporidiosis.

treatment relies on supportive oral fluid therapy, administered under veterinary guidance. Oocysts can survive for long periods in the environment, and are resistant to most disinfectants, so prevention depends on strict hygiene and the regular movement of susceptible lambs to a cleaner environment.

Neonatal Salmonellosis

Outbreaks of salmonellosis in lambs are rare, and usually follow the purchase of infected carrier sheep or calves. Most cases are caused by *Salmonella typhimurium* or *Salmonella Dublin*, although exotic salmonellae have been reported. *S. Dublin* infection is usually associated with cattle, while *S. typhimurium* is not host-specific. Most *Salmonella* species are potentially zoonotic.

Salmonella bacteria cause severe intestinal inflammation, destroying the absorptive capacity and stimulating secretion. They are also invasive, leading to bacteraemia and infection of other organ systems. The clinical signs are weakness and profuse green-brown coloured, blood-stained, foetid-smelling diarrhoea, with variable levels of elevation of body temperature (pyrexia), dehydration and breathing difficulty (dyspnoea). The disease rapidly progresses to recumbency and death. The success of treatment of affected lambs with intensive fluid therapy, broad spectrum systemic antibiotics and NSAIDs is variable. Lambs which recover are ill-thrifty and may be carriers.

Enteric Viruses

Rotavirus and coronavirus infections do not appear to cause primary disease in lambs, although lambs may be infected during the first week of life. These infections invade small intestinal villous epithelial cells, causing villous atrophy and compensatory crypt cell proliferation, and resulting in decreased absorption and increased secretion. The main role of enteric viruses in causing disease is to enable the establishment of other enteric infections, such as cryptosporidiosis.

Hepatic Necrobacillosis

Navel infection with *Fusobacterium necrophorum* can result in the formation of abscesses in the liver and secondary spread to joints and lungs (Figure 2.13). Most outbreaks of necrobacillosis are associated with poor environmental hygiene and poor passive immunity.

Clinical signs are typically seen in lambs 10–20 days old, and are characterised by ill thrift and a hunch-backed stance. The response to antibiotic and anti-inflammatory treatment is poor, again emphasising the importance of hygiene and early colostrum intake in disease prevention.

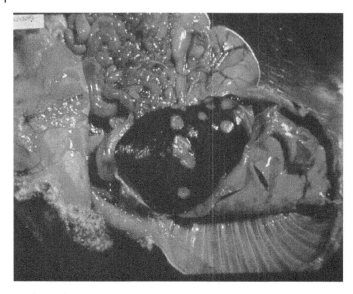

Figure 2.13 Post-mortem image showing multiple abscesses in the liver and lungs caused by *Fusobacterium necrophorum* bacteria. The bacteria entered the body through the navel, then spread to the liver and then to the lungs, via the portal blood circulation. Identification of multiple cases of hepatic necrobacillosis generally indicates poor standards of hygiene in the lambing environment.

Neonatal Bacteraemias (joint ill, navel ill, endocarditis and meningitis)

Most cases of joint ill, navel ill, endocarditis or meningitis occur in colostrum-deprived lambs, following systemic invasion via the tonsils or gut of a range of opportunistic pathogenic bacteria acquired from a heavily contaminated environment.

Joint ill (polyarthritis) is sometimes seen in lambs as young as five days old, although clinical signs are not usually seen until 2–3 weeks old (Figure 2.14). Affected lambs are lame, with severe pain, heat and swelling of multiple limb joints, as well as reduced sucking behaviour which cause ill thrift. The response to antibiotic and anti-inflammatory drug treatment is generally poor, so the emphasis should be placed on preventive management.

Streptococcus dysgalactiae is a common cause of polyarthritis in lambs less than four weeks old. In the acute stages of the disease, lambs are stiff or weak, but affected joints are not generally distended. Joint enlargement due to the accumulation of pus only appears as a chronic feature. Lambs may acquire infection from the teats or milk of a carrier ewe, but *S. dysgalactiae* survives well on dry straw and wool, so a source of infection may be from a heavily contaminated environment. High numbers of lambs are sometimes affected, despite good hygiene and colostrum management. Treatment with high doses of penicillin and corticosteroids is generally successful when cases are recognised early.

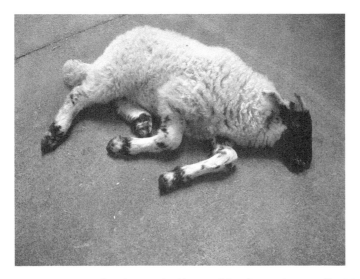

Figure 2.14 Joint ill is characterised by painful and sometimes swollen joints in the limbs or spinal column.

Spinal abscesses are diagnosed sporadically in lambs 4–12 weeks old, following bacterial spread from another focus of infection via blood vessels. Most cases involve *Trueperella pyogenes* or *Staphylococcus aureus* bacteria. Spinal abscesses may also occasionally arise following trauma, or from the spread of infection from docking wounds. The clinical signs depend on the location of the abscess and the degree of spinal cord compression. Signs are often sudden in onset in otherwise healthy lambs. Lesions involving the cervical vertebral column are characterised by paralysis and weakness involving all four limbs, while lower cervical and lumbar lesions cause flaccidity of the thoracic limbs and spasticity of the pelvic limbs. Affected lambs often adopt a dog-sitting position. Most cases require euthanasia to prevent further suffering.

Navel infection occurs as a sequel to neonatal bacteraemia, or directly from a contaminated environment. Affected lambs adopt a hunch-backed stance, show poor sucking behaviour, develop a hollow flanked appearance and lose weight (Figure 2.15). Affected navels are moist, swollen and painful, and sometimes exude pus. Abdominal palpation sometimes demonstrates painful internal swelling extending to the liver. The response to antibiotic and anti-inflammatory drug treatment depends on the extent and duration of infection.

Meningoencephalitis occurs sporadically in 4–6 week old lambs. The early clinical signs include a lack of a sucking reflex, with abnormal ocular reflexes, weakness and an altered gait. As the disease progresses, lambs develop signs of depression, leading to stupor, and become hyperaesthetic, overreacting to auditory and tactile stimuli. Affected lambs are often recumbent, with their pelvic limbs extended and their neck flexed backwards (Figure 2.16). Seizures are observed during the terminal stages of the disease.

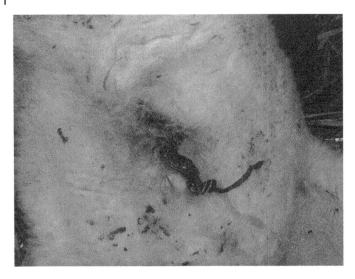

Figure 2.15 Typical appearance of a swollen navel.

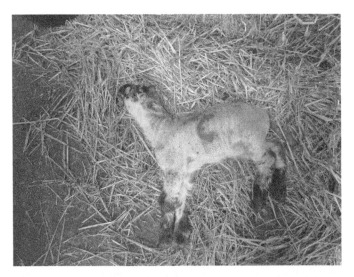

Figure 2.16 Extension of the pelvic limbs and backward flexion of the neck of a lamb due to meningoencephalitis.

The treatment response to corticosteroids and high doses of antibiotics is poor. Prevention depends on ensuring adequate early passive antibody transfer through colostrum, and maintaining a hygienic environment.

To summarise, correct maternal nutrition, control of abortion and the prevention of dystocia are essential to ensure optimal physiological adaptation of the newborn lamb to extra-uterine life. Management practices to further minimise the prevalence of neonatal bacteraemias are shown in Table 2.1.

Table 2.1 Specific management to minimise the impact of joint ill, navel ill, and meningitis in lambs.

Availability of sufficient skilled assistants to monitor all neonatal lambs, to detect and investigate disease and instigate early treatment.

Installation of good access to lambing pens and good lighting.

A compact lambing period to maximise the use of labour and minimise the potential for build-up of disease in the lambing environment.

Maintenance of strict hygiene in lambing accommodation. In the case of housed ewes, it is important that both the lambing courts and individual pens are kept clean, to minimise contamination of ewes' fleeces and udders. Buildings should be well ventilated and drained. Individual pens should be well lit, easily accessible and cleaned between occupants. Ewe lambs and long-tailed ewes should be dagged prior to entering lambing accommodation. Daily application of paraformaldehyde granules to the bedding can prove to be helpful.

The stocking rate of housed lambing accommodation should not exceed one ewe per $1.1\,m^2$, and the area of individual pens should be at least $3.0\,m^2$. Provision of one individual pen per eight housed ewes is recommended.

Dipping all lambs' navels in strong iodine solution at birth and again, ideally, four hours later.

Ensuring that all lambs receive adequate colostrum within the first four hours of life. If in doubt, administer 50 ml/kg of colostrum or colostrum substitute by stomach tube.

Ensuring that hot water and a full clean lambing kit is easily available.

Checking all penned lambs regularly for signs of brightness and full stomachs. Navels should be brittle within 36 hours of birth.

Navel Dipping of Lambs

The navels of all lambs should be treated as soon as possible after birth. Tincture of iodine (10%) is the preferred product. The use of oxytetracycline spray is inferior, as this does not dry the tissue and causes the umbilical cord to shrivel up, leaving it as a portal for infection. The best way to apply tincture of iodine is using a teat dip cup to immerse the navel completely, coating all surfaces (Figure 2.17). Ideally, navels should be treated three times at six-hour intervals, particularly if there is a problem with septicaemia, joint ill or navel ill on the farm.

Floppy Kid and Drunken Lamb Syndromes

Floppy kid and the rarer drunken lamb syndromes are metabolic disturbances that affect young kids and lambs, usually between 4–11 days old. Signs include weakness, inability to suck, lack of appetite, a sleepy appearance and bending of the front legs (Figure 2.18). Affected animals do not scour, are not dehydrated, and are not fevered. A bloated and distended abdomen and excessive salivation may develop. The disease is caused by a metabolic acidosis, and animals recover once this is corrected. Treatment options include intravenous administration of sodium bicarbonate solution (65 ml of 1.3% solution or 16 ml of 5% solution per kg body weight) or oral administration of sodium bicarbonate (0.84 g per kg body weight dissolved in 30–100 ml water and administered by stomach tube).

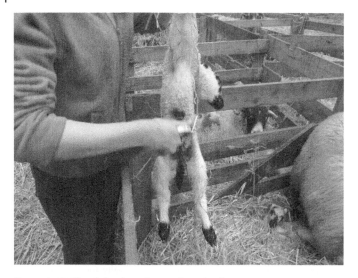

Figure 2.17 Navel dipping of a newborn lamb.

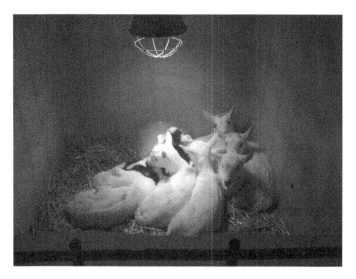

Figure 2.18 Floppy kid syndrome is a common cause of weakness between 4 and 11 days old. These kids are being kept in clean and comfortable conditions in an attempt to avoid the problem.

Trace Element and Mineral Deficiencies Affecting Newborn Lambs

Iodine deficiency is an occasional cause of high mortality rates in newborn lambs and kids (Figure 2.19). Most problems are caused by grazing late pregnant ewes on pastures or crops containing high levels of thiocyanate goitrogens. Thiocyanates act as goitrogens by blocking the uptake of inorganic iodine by the thyroid gland. Their goitrogenic effect is largely overcome by iodine supplementation.

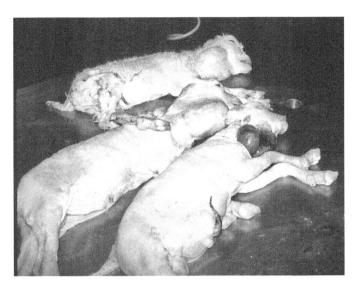

Figure 2.19 Newborn goat kids with severe goitre. These cases often indicate the presence of other, less severely affected animals in the herd.

The most obvious clinical sign of iodine deficiency is goitre in newborn lambs. Lambs with congenital goitre may be pot-bellied in appearance and have scant wool, which lacks crimp. Lambs from the same litter can be affected to different extremes. Animals with severe goitre usually die soon after birth.

Subclinical iodine deficiency sometimes results in high perinatal lamb mortality rates in flocks where clinical goitre is not diagnosed. Typically, high lamb losses occur during adverse weather conditions, due to starvation and hypothermia, or stillbirths where the foetal membranes still cover the lamb's nose. This is due to the role of iodine in thyroid hormones in foetal maturation and thermoregulation.

Swayback in young lambs occurs as a consequence of severe copper deficiency in mid-to-late pregnant ewes. Most outbreaks of swayback have been seen following mild winters when little supplementary feeding was provided during mid-pregnancy.

Congenital swayback is characterised by stillbirths and the birth of small and weak lambs, which may show fine tremors of the head. Less severely affected lambs are bright but uncoordinated, with characteristic weakness of the pelvic limbs, which results in a swaying or stumbling gait. These lambs are often fine-boned and dull-coated. A delayed form of the disease, with slow, progressive weakness and muscle atrophy of the pelvic limbs, is occasionally seen in older lambs, sometimes initiated by gathering or handling (Figure 2.20).

Historically, nutritional muscular dystrophy was an important common selenium responsive cause of perinatal lamb mortality in sheep flocks. The disease is now uncommon, due to awareness of selenium deficiency and widespread supplementation.

The disease in lambs is congenital, or delayed in onset. Congenital disease results in stillbirths or the birth of weak lambs, which fail to feed and die from

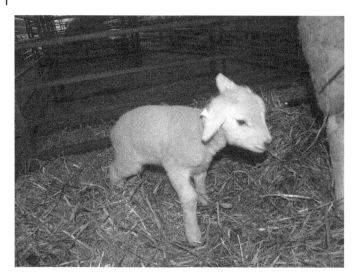

Figure 2.20 A lamb with swayback. Similar clinical signs must be differentiated from those of other common problems, such as spinal abscess.

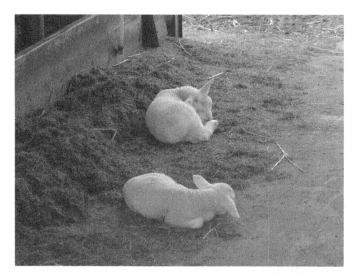

Figure 2.21 Clinical signs of white muscle disease must be differentiated from those of other common problems causing weakness, in order to avoid unhelpfully wrong diagnoses.

starvation. The delayed onset disease is also been reported in lambs after docking. Clinical signs appear suddenly, and are usually precipitated by exercise and stress such as docking, bad weather or transport. Affected animals show sudden-onset semi-flaccid paralysis, but appear stiff or unable to stand (Figure 2.21). Lambs show difficulty in sucking, due to pharyngeal paralysis, so may die from starvation and/or hypothermia. Some lambs are found dead as a result of respiratory failure. Surviving animals are ill-thrifty.

Congenital Malformations of Newborn Lambs

A very low incidence of congenital lamb deformities (such as: limb malformations; defects of the urinary tract; genital abnormalities; undershot lower jaw (mandible) and lengthening of the upper jaw (maxilla); overshot mandible; failure of closure of vessels between the navel and bladder (persistent urachus); umbilical herniation; atresia ani; eye abnormalities; micrencephaly; schistosoma reflexa; and spina bifida) is seen in most sheep flocks and goat herds, caused by random genetic mutations and developmental anomalies. Lambs with potentially fatal malformations are sometimes born alive, and require euthanasia immediately after birth. Some malformations, such as undershot jaw and genital abnormalities, are not fatal, but result in ill thrift in affected animals.

Rare large-scale outbreaks of congenital malformations may be associated with foetal exposure to viruses, such as border disease virus, or toxins.

Congenital malformations of lambs may be associated with genetic disease resulting from random unfavourable recombinations and expression of abnormal genes. Most heritable genetic diseases are recessive, or show incomplete penetrance in their expression, and are affected by other genetic, phenotypic and environmental influences. Genetic disease is insidious and may be present in large numbers of animals, and is therefore difficult to control before clinical signs are first recognised.

Entropion

Entropion is a common congenital disorder, which is characterised by turning in of one or both lower eyelids (Figure 2.22). The condition is seen in most breeds of sheep and is probably inherited, but the nature of the inheritance is unknown. In-turned hairs of the lower eyelid rub on the cornea and cause severe irritation. The condition is painful, and affected eyes appear half-closed and watery. Some cases spontaneously recover but in most lambs, unless treated, the cornea becomes cloudy and ulcerated, leading to permanent blindness.

Mildly affected cases often respond to manual turning out (eversion) of the lower eyelid (Figure 2.23). Lambs should be carefully monitored afterwards and the procedure may need to be repeated.

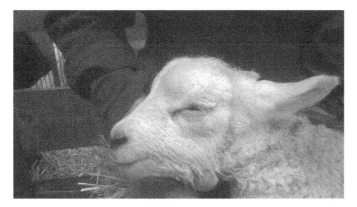

Figure 2.22 Turning in of a lower eyelid (entropion) is a painful condition in lambs.

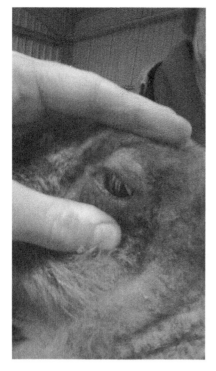

Figure 2.23 Manual eversion of an in-turned lower eyelid.

More severely affected eyes are usually treated by injection of about 1 ml of penicillin under the eyelid (Figure 2.24). The lamb is securely restrained, and a thumb of one hand is used to roll the eyelid forwards while using the other hand to insert a one-inch 21 g needle under the eyelid from the outside, so that the tip points towards the lamb's nose. The penicillin is then injected under the conjunctiva.

Alternatively, metal (Michel) clips can be applied just below the eyelid, to gather and tense loose skin and draw the eyelid outwards (Figure 2.25). Severe or persistent cases sometimes require local analgesia and surgical removal of a strip of skin from under the eyelid (Figure 2.26).

Atresia Ani

Lambs are sometimes born with a developmental abnormality, resulting in an inperforate anus. After a few days,

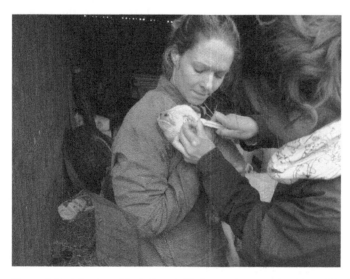

Figure 2.24 Injection of 1 ml of penicillin beneath the conjunctiva of the lower eye.

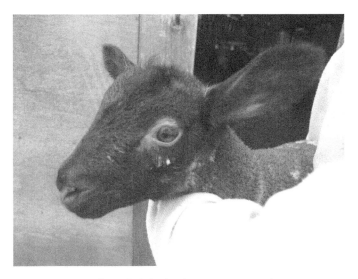

Figure 2.25 Use of a Michel clip for the management of entropion.

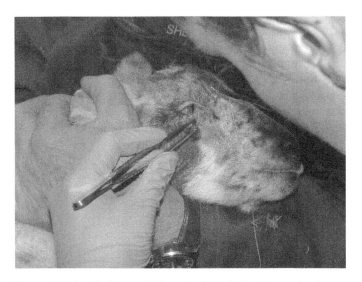

Figure 2.26 Surgical removal of a strip of skin below the eye for the treatment of persistent cases of entropion should only be undertaken by a vet.

these lambs develop distended abdomens and become uncomfortable (Figure 2.27). Some cases, where the position of the anus is apparent because of pressure in the rectum beneath, respond well to surgical correction. Surgery involves making a simple cross-shaped skin incision over the bulging rectum where the anus should have been. In some cases, the distal rectum is also absent, and corrective surgery is not possible.

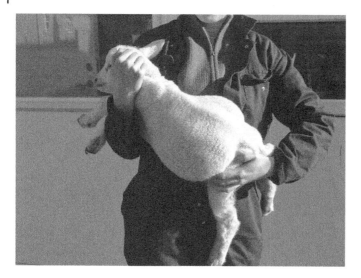

Figure 2.27 Massive abdominal distension resulting from atresia ani. Lambs are sometimes two weeks old before the clinical signs are noted.

Umbilical Hernia

The umbilicus forms a gap in the body wall in the navel region, through which blood vessels from the placenta gained access to the foetus' circulation through the navel cord. This gap normally closes soon after birth but, occasionally, does not, either due to a congenital defect or due to trauma. The gap may remain big enough to allow the abdominal contents to be herniated. Most cases are identified once the small intestines have been herniated (Figure 2.28). The problem is exacerbated by the ewe's persistent licking.

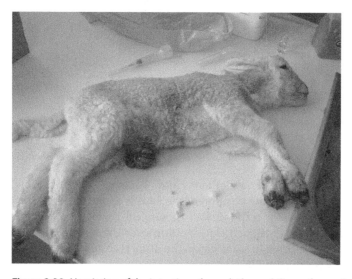

Figure 2.28 Herniation of the intestines through the umbilicus of a newborn lamb.

If identified early, and in the absence to trauma to the intestines, it is possible to replace and surgically repair the hernia. This is an act of veterinary medicine, and can only be performed by a veterinary surgeon. For repair to be successful, the herniated organs must be kept clean, moist and free from further traumatic damage. If the intestines are already heavily contaminated or damaged, immediate euthanasia is required.

Lamb Losses Subsequent to the Neonatal Period

The majority of lambs which die between one week old and weaning do so as a result of disease acquired during the perinatal period. Significant losses sometimes occur due to specific diseases, such pasteurellosis, *Erysipelothrix rhusiopathiae* polyarthritis, nephrosis, coccidiosis and nematodirosis, which are acquired after one week of age.

Significant losses occasionally occur due to exposure. Healthy lambs can withstand severe weather, although blizzard conditions can overcome this resilience. Losses to exposure are particularly distressing as, in many cases, there is little that can be done to prevent them. Provision of shelter and use of safe areas can help, but this requires considerable skill and knowledge of the environment to implement. Many sheep have been lost while seeking shelter in areas subsequently filled by snow drifts.

Limb Fractures

Broken legs occur occasionally in lambs or kids on most farms, following accidents or misadventure. It is important to recognise these cases promptly, and to manage them appropriately. Fractures above or through the hock or carpus, those with multiple fragments, or those where the bone has penetrated the skin, do not generally heal well. In these cases, immediate consideration must be given to preventing further pain and suffering. Simple breaks of the lower limb not involving the joint can be amenable to treatment by casting or splinting.

The lamb must be gently, but firmly, restrained. Consideration must be given to the fact that any manipulation of the fracture is painful, and must be undertaken skilfully, otherwise veterinary assistance must be sought. This usually involves restrained use of traction to pull the broken ends of the bone apart before realigning them. Next, a layer of padding should be placed around the leg. This should be thick enough to be effective, but not so thick as to loosen the splint or cast. Next, the splint(s) or cast is applied. When using splints, it is important to prevent movement of the fracture site in all directions. Splints can be secured using sticky tape, material or cord (Figure 2.29). Casts should be applied according to the manufacturer's instructions (Figure 2.30).

Following splinting or casting, the lamb should be able to walk. The splints or cast should not be too heavy, which might prevent the lamb lifting the limb, or too tight, so as to cut off the blood supply, or too loose, which might not immobilise the fracture or could cause chafing. Splints should be removed and

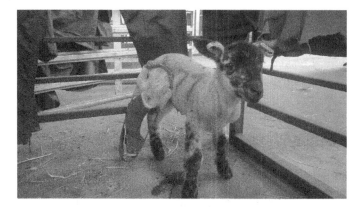

Figure 2.29 Use of splints to immobilise a broken limb.

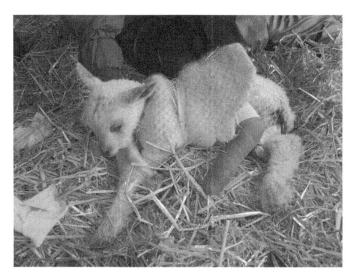

Figure 2.30 Use of a cast to immobilise a broken limb.

reapplied every two weeks in growing lambs. Casts should be left for no more than three weeks. Most fractures in young lambs and kids heal in 3–4 weeks. It is not unusual to have a bony swelling at the site of fracture healing, but this should be stable and non-painful.

Lambs and kids with splints or casts should be able to follow their mothers and suckle in an enclosed space, such as a clean, dry shed or small paddock; however, they should not be put out into an open field. Any such lambs spending excessive time lying down should be re-examined, to check the limb and detect any other problems.

3

Husbandry and Health Planning to Prepare for Lambing or Kidding: Ensuring Pregnancy in Ewes and Does

There is a perception amongst many small ruminant farmers and keepers that lambing or kidding represents the beginning of the annual flock or herd management calendar. Consequently, efforts aimed at ensuring a basis for optimal flock or herd production and welfare often begin with the management of parturient ewes or does and their lambs or kids, making lambing or kidding the busiest and most stressful time of year.

However, a more efficient approach involves the concept of lambing or kidding being part of a continuum of sheep or goat husbandry, the outcome of which is determined by flock or herd management, and interventions occurring throughout the year. Thus, the foundations for a successful lambing or kidding period are laid long beforehand, during the approach to the mating period. This chapter describes reproductive management, nutrition and disease control, with regards to the requirements for reproduction and mating management.

Reproductive Management

The Breeding Season

Sheep and goats are more or less incapable of breeding for a large part of the year, and undergo repeated reproductive cycles during the breeding season until they become pregnant (described as being seasonally polyoestrous).

The oestrous cycle starts and ends with the release of eggs capable of being fertilised (ovulation), and is about 17 days long in sheep. Ovulation is accompanied by behavioural changes known as 'oestrus' or 'heat'. During oestrus, ewes are both attractive and receptive to rams. Ewes will seek out a ram and may adopt a crouching posture, while displaying tail wagging or nuzzling the ram's flank before standing to be mated. Oestrus lasts for approximately 36 hours in sheep, and ovulation occurs 18–24 hours after it begins. The first oestrus of the season is often described as being silent, whereby ewes display no behavioural signs. Ewe lambs often have slightly shorter oestrous cycles than mature ewes, and frequently do not display overt oestrous behaviour; hence, the general advice that they should be mated by experienced rams of high libido.

Practical Lambing and Lamb Care – A Veterinary Guide, Fourth Edition.
Neil Sargison, James Patrick Crilly and Andrew Hopker.
© 2018 John Wiley & Sons Ltd. Published 2018 by John Wiley & Sons Ltd.

Onset of the breeding season in sheep is driven by short day length. Sheep are short-day breeders so, for most breeds originating from northerly latitudes, the natural mating period is in autumn. Coupled with a pregnancy of about 145 days (about five months), this naturally results in lambs being born in the spring, coinciding with fresh herbage growth that provides sufficient nutrition to support the high energy demands of late pregnancy and lactation.

Certain sheep breeds originating from equatorial latitudes have much longer breeding seasons. The physiological mechanism governing the onset of the breeding season is the release of a hormone called melatonin from the pineal gland region of the brain during the hours of darkness. As the day length decreases, melatonin release increases, indirectly stimulating release of the hormones which control the reproductive cycle, resulting in a return of fertility. The breeding season is defined as starting once all healthy ewes are cycling, following a transitional period when a few are cycling. In fact, the majority can be induced to cycle during the transitional period, using synthetic reproductive hormones. Rams are likewise affected by the change in day length, with testicular size, sperm production and libido peaking in the autumn. There are breed differences in the length of the breeding season, characterised by more northerly and mountain breeds having a shorter breeding season than lowland breeds, although variation between breeds can be significant.

Breed Selection with Reference to Reproduction and Lamb Care

The choice of appropriate dam and sire breeds is an important part of the preparation for lambing. Breed selection is also important with reference to other key performance indicators, such as carcase conformation, lamb growth, or milk yields.

Breeds should be appropriate for particular management systems and environments. For example, hardy, easy-lambing breeds such as the Swaledale, Cheviot, Shetland or Scottish Blackface are more appropriate for outdoor lambing with minimal intervention (Figure 3.1) than more prolific ewe breeds producing large lambs.

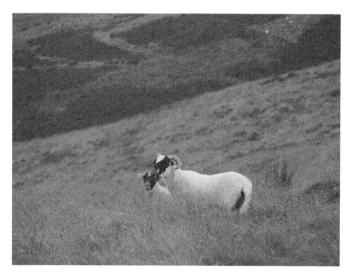

Figure 3.1 Scottish Blackface ewes are well suited to the harsh conditions in which they are kept.

Table 3.1 Breed selection criteria with reference to lambing management.

Characteristic	Relevance
Length of the breeding period	Earlier lambing is possible for breeds with longer breeding periods. Longer breeding periods allow the better use of reproductive manipulation within the transition period.
Litter size	Selection for large litter sizes can improve production and profitability, but increases the risk of lamb losses unless accompanied by appropriate nutrition and lambing management.
Mothering ability	Under lambing systems involving minimal intervention, the ewes' mothering ability must be good in order to minimise the risk of lamb abandonment and subsequent lamb losses from hypothermia and/or starvation.
Hardiness	Sheep kept on extensive grazing, where they are exposed to adverse weather and potentially restricted nutrition, must be hardy to cope with, and avoid loss of, ewes and lambs.
Pelvic conformation	Pelvic conformation varies between and within breeds. Ewes with narrow or unnaturally angled pelvises have a high risk of requiring assistance at lambing, and hence require intensive supervision.

However, mountain breeds, with short breeding seasons, slow growth rates and relatively poor carcase conformation, would be a poor choice for early lambing indoors in January with the aim of producing lamb meat for the Easter market, compared with lowland breeds such as the Suffolk or Dorset. Characteristics which should be considered when selecting appropriate breeds with relevance to lambing management are shown in Table 3.1.

Rams contribute 50% of the genetic make-up of a flock's lamb output. However, what may be desirable characteristics in the mother may not be so in the offspring if they are intended for different purposes. Hence, the paternal genetic contribution must also be considered to produce optimal offspring, without compromising the important characteristics of the ewe flock (Figure 3.2).

Selection of Animals for Culling

Selection of ewes for removal from the breeding flock should be a continuous process with the aims of:

i) removing unhealthy animals which are not productive;
ii) removal of ewes with defects or poor production traits that may be passed on to their lambs; and
iii) removal of ewes whose management necessitates inputs that are out of proportion to their contribution to flock production.

These aims often overlap. For example, chronically lame sheep are likely to be in poor condition, so are not as fecund as, or produce less milk than, their sound counterparts. These poorly productive animals require repeated and often

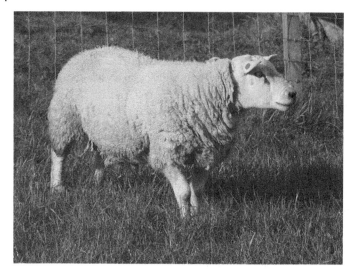

Figure 3.2 Terminal sire rams such as the Texel breed are suited to the production of fast-growing lambs with good carcase conformation.

unsuccessful treatment to alleviate their suffering, and their lameness may have a heritable component, as in the case of poor limb conformation. Thus, the decision to cull chronically lame ewes is based on a range of voluntary and involuntary considerations.

Various reasons for culling are first identified in pregnant and lambing ewes. However, it is usually inappropriate to cull these animals before weaning. Consequently, problems arising at lambing should be recorded, and ewes identified and marked for subsequent consideration. Examples of common periparturient problems that should be considered as reasons for culling are given in Table 3.2.

Weaning is an opportunity to examine the entire ewe flock and select animals for culling (Figure 3.3).

Additional factors to consider at weaning are shown in Table 3.3. Weaning also affords an opportunity to assess disease levels across the flock as a whole, while most of the ewes and lambs are present. Lameness levels, evidence of previous mastitis and average body condition scores all give valuable information on the general flock health status. Where a flock has a known problem with untreatable chronic diseases, such as maedi-visna, Johne's disease, ovine pulmonary adeno-carcinoma (jaagsiekte) and caseous lypmphadenitis, specific culling policies to minimise the spread and impact of these diseases on productivity should be implemented.

In the absence of a flock-wide or a ram-specific breeding soundness problem, 2% or fewer ewes bred within the breeding season should be barren after a mating period spanning two reproductive cycles. Such ewes may be incapable of breeding, or they may have inherently poor natural fertility. Hence, retaining

Table 3.2 Common periparturient problems for consideration as reasons for culling ewes.

Problem	Decision	Reason
Vaginal prolapse	Cull	Affected animals are more likely to prolapse in subsequent years.
Uterine prolapse	Cull or retain	Often occurs in young or old ewes in poor body condition, or associated with hypocalcaemia. Recurrence is unlikely once predisposing causes are managed.
Difficult lambing (dystocia) due to foetal malpresentation	Retain	The problem is most likely to have arisen due to management factors, and is unlikely to be directly heritable.
Dystocia due to failure of cervical dilation (ringwomb)	Cull	The problem may be heritable or may be a result of previous scarring of the cervix. It is likely to recur in subsequent years.
Dystocia due to poor pelvic conformation	Cull	The problem is related to the genetic makeup of the ewe.
Dystocia due to foetal oversize	Cull or retain	If the problem is due to maternal factors, culling is advised; however, if due to excessive nutrition or inappropriate choice of sire, it can be avoided in subsequent years.
Ewe requiring Caesarean section	Cull or retain	The reason for the ewe requiring Caesarean section should be considered. Some fail to re-breed.
Poor mothering behaviour	Cull or retain	Ewes showing poor mothering ability in extensive management systems should be culled. Under more intensive systems, the problem may be a result of inexperience or inappropriate management.
Mastitis	Cull	Udder damage will inevitably result in poor milk production in subsequent lactations.
Poor milk production	Cull or retain	If poor milk production is an individual animal problem, the affected ewe should be culled. If it is a flock problem, the cause may be nutritional and remedied in subsequent years. Check for mastitis before retaining.
Hypocalcaemia (milk fever)	Retain	The problem is related to stress and nutritional management.
Hypomagnesaemia (staggers)	Retain	The problem is related to stress and nutritional management.
Pregnancy toxaemia	Retain	The problem is related to large litter size and nutritional management.
Pre-pubic tendon rupture (ventral hernia)	Cull	The rupture will not repair.

them and their offspring potentially lowers the average fertility of the flock, reducing productivity. These non-productive ewes should be identified as early as possible, for example at ultrasound scanning for pregnancy, and then removed from the flock.

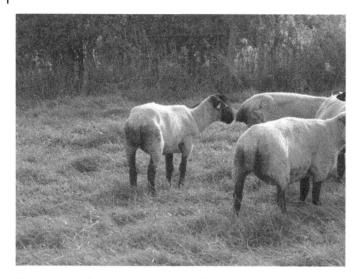

Figure 3.3 Involuntary culling resulting from poor animal health must be kept to a minimum through planned management, allowing for flock genetic improvement through voluntary culling of less productive animals.

Table 3.3 Additional considerations for culling ewes at weaning.

Body condition	Body condition score all sheep. Too low a score across the flock suggests a disease or management problem. Small numbers of thin ewes may be given access to better grazing or supplementary feeding. Very thin ewes and those which fail to improve should be culled.
Teeth	Ewes with missing or broken front teeth will find it harder to maintain condition on short grazing. Depending on severity, they may be managed separately or culled. Ewes with abnormal cheek teeth should be culled.
Udder	The udder should be palpated for evidence of mastitis, such as hard swellings, or discharging tracts. Ewes with evidence of mastitis should be culled.
Feet	Lame ewes struggle to maintain body condition. Ewes with uncomplicated or early infectious causes should be treated as appropriate. Ewes which remain lame despite treatment should be culled. Ewes with deformed feet, misshapen limbs or swelling of the joints should be culled, as they are unlikely to recover.

Selection of Replacement Breeding Ewes

Breeding replacements may be mated to lamb at either one year old (ewe lambs), or at two years old (referred to as yearlings, two-tooths, or gimmers). In some flocks, breeding replacements may have been bred previously (for example, purchased as cast hill or upland ewes). All breeding replacements should be subjected to an examination similar to that performed on ewes at weaning. Where cast ewes are purchased as breeding replacements, the vulva should also be checked for evidence of scarring from retention sutures used for vaginal prolapses.

Whenever possible, purchased replacements should be sourced from flocks of equal or higher health status, and should undergo a quarantine period and protocol devised in conjunction with the farm's veterinary health plan.

As ewe lambs and gimmers have not lambed before, the likelihood of mastitis changes to the udder is low. A low tolerance should be shown towards poor body condition, because these animals have not experienced the high protein and energy demands of previous lactation. Replacements should have good general body conformation. Where replacements are homebred, they can be selected on the basis of performance as lambs (for example, having stood quickly, sucked quickly and grown rapidly), as well as on maternal performance (for example, preferentially retaining the offspring of ewes which lamb and successfully rear twins every year). Offspring of ewes identified as suffering from Johne's disease, maedi-visna or ovine pulmonary adenocarcinoma (jaagsiekte) should not be kept as replacements, as the close contact between ewe and lamb means that the lambs may be infected.

The decision to breed replacement females for the first time as lambs or yearlings is not straightforward. Breeding as ewe lambs has the advantage that unproductive animals do not need to be kept for an entire year. However, the system requires careful planning and meticulous attention to detail in order to avoid disappointing fertility and fecundity, unsatisfactory levels of lambing intervention, poor lamb survival, retarded growth, loss of maternal body condition and poor fertility during the following year. Breeding as yearlings also requires good management, but is a more forgiving system.

Ewe lambs must achieve at least 60% of their expected mature bodyweight at mating, and should be in good body condition (score 3.0–3.5 on a five-point scale). Ewe lambs that are thinner or smaller than this will have reduced ovulation rates and poorer milk production. Unlike the situation when feeding pregnant yearlings and adult ewes – where provision must be made for maintenance, foetal growth and lactation – when feeding pregnant ewe lambs, the additional requirements for their own growth must also be considered.

Ram Breeding Soundness Examination

Rams should be examined about three months before the start of the mating period. This allows adequate time for correction of problems, or for culling and sourcing replacements.

Rams should be in good body condition, but not fat at mating (score 3.5–4.0 on a five-point scale). Good limb and mouth conformation is important in rams, both due to their contribution to the genetic make-up of their lambs, and because animals with poor conformation may become lame or thin and, hence, may not remain sound and active throughout the mating period. Rams should be checked for tooth abnormalities, visual impairment, lameness and brisket sores, each of which can reduce their breeding soundness (Figure 3.4).

The rams' scrotal contents should be palpated (Figure 3.5). The testes should be freely mobile within the scrotum, evenly sized and have an even, slightly yielding feel. Testicular size is correlated with potential for sperm production. This can be judged by gently pressing the testes into the bottom of the scrotum, using a hand applied around the scrotal neck, and then measuring the circumference of the scrotum at its widest point. Most mature rams should have a scrotal circumference at its widest point between 30–40 cm. Outside the breeding season,

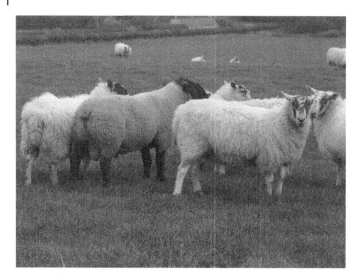

Figure 3.4 Rams need to be physically sound as well as being reproductively sound.

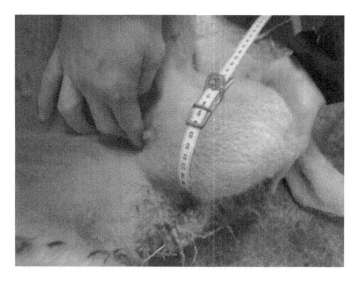

Figure 3.5 Palpation of a ram's scrotal contents can be conducted with the animal standing, or cast onto its hindquarters. Sargison 2008. Reproduced with permission of John Wiley and Sons.

the scrotal contents will shrink and be less firm, but at no point should they be widely different in size, or of variable texture.

The tails and heads of the epididymes, where sperm matures and is stored after production in the testes, are easily palpated below and above the testes. These should be attached to the testis, albeit with a clear boundary. They should feel firm and smooth, but not swollen or painful, and there should be no discharging tracts (Figure 3.6).

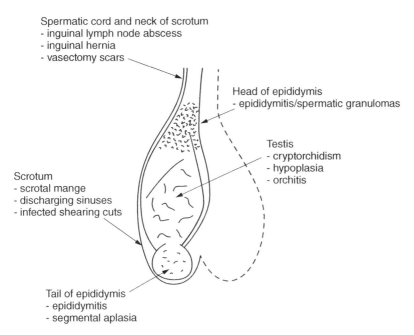

Spermatic cord and neck of scrotum
- inguinal lymph node abscess
- inguinal hernia
- vasectomy scars

Head of epididymis
- epididymitis/spermatic granulomas

Testis
- cryptorchidism
- hypoplasia
- orchitis

Scrotum
- scrotal mange
- discharging sinuses
- infected shearing cuts

Tail of epididymis
- epididymitis
- segmental aplasia

Figure 3.6 Diagrammatic representation of what is palpated during ram breeding soundness examination. Sargison 2008. Reproduced with permission of John Wiley and Sons.

A purple-coloured flush of the skin of the inner thigh occurs during the breeding season, reflecting elevated testosterone levels. The scrotal skin should be thin and supple. The scrotum and its contents should hang well below the body of the standing ram, providing a cooling effect that aids sperm production and maturation. Any thickening or inflammation of the scrotum can result in an elevated temperature in the scrotum, and may impair sperm production.

The penis can be extruded by grasping it firmly at its base while the ram is restrained on his rump. The penis should not be attached to the prepuce (sheath), and there should be no obviously abnormal swellings, inflammation or discharge.

Electroejaculation and ram examination must not be performed routinely, but may be helpful only in cases where an individual has been identified as having poor or suspect reproductive performance, yet clear abnormalities have not been found on physical examination. The procedure may only be performed by a veterinary surgeon. In some cases, ultrasound examination of the scrotal contents can be a useful adjunct in the diagnosis of abnormalities.

Selection of Replacement Rams

Replacement rams should have no detectable abnormalities on breeding soundness examination. They should have a large scrotal circumference relative to their age and time of year. They should also have good body conformation and general health. Consideration must be given to good biosecurity and disease control.

Rams should not be introduced into tick-infested areas from areas with no ticks. This is to avoid the risks of tick-borne diseases which can affect breeding soundness, such as tick-borne fever, occurring in the naïve introduced animals.

Care must be taken to ensure that home-bred replacement rams are not used on their own relatives. Home-bred rams should be selected on the basis of recorded data for their vigour as neonates, growth rates, health and performance in the face of disease challenges. Where the dam's breeding history is known, those rams whose mothers who have performed favourably, for example showing good mothering ability, should be preferentially selected.

Biosecurity

Effective biosecurity to prevent the introduction of new diseases or problems necessitates:

- isolation and quarantine;
- assessment of the risk of introduction of specific problems;
- appropriate treatments on arrival;
- sourcing animals from flocks with similar or higher status for freedom from specific diseases; and
- preventing diseases in the introduced animals that are already endemic in the main flock.

The period of time for which animals are kept in quarantine should be sufficient to allow them to be clinically examined for the presence of disease (for example, footrot or contagious ovine digital dermatitis) and successfully treated as required. The threat of introduction of anthelmintic resistant nematodes is always present, so animals should be treated with a combination of anthelmintic drugs that is likely to be effective against resistant parasites on arrival. Effective treatments to remove sheep scab mites and anthelmintic resistant liver flukes should be given, depending on the risk assessment. Knowledge of the disease-freedom status of source flocks depends on the availability and understanding of the use of diagnostic tests – for example, used in the Premium Health Scheme for chlamydial abortion in the UK. Control of endemic diseases might involve vaccination and strategic treatments.

Breeding Replacement Selection Policies

There is a great deal of between breed and within flock variation as regards many traits. Some of this variation is acquired and some has a genetic basis, but the majority of traits are influenced by both factors. For example, the milk production of an individual ewe is dependent on the adequacy of nutrition during lactation, prior effects of the diet on udder development as a ewe lamb, and damage caused by mastitis and current demands, as well as her genetic potential.

Selection for production traits is possible, but only improves economic productivity when the animals' environment and management are appropriate. For example, it is pointless trying to breed ewes for genetically greater milk production if their diet fails to provide sufficient nutrients to allow them to produce

Table 3.4 Steps in the genetic selection process for production traits.

Identification of the trait(s) for selection	Selecting for several traits at once results in slower progress than selecting for one single trait. Some traits respond better to selection than do others.
Scoring of animals for production traits	Good record-keeping is important to identify animals with desirable traits and take into account the performance of their relatives.
Selection of animals	The more heavily a trait is selected for, the more quickly a population average shift is seen. Removing the bottom 5% each year may rid the flock of problem animals, but will probably not shift the average. Removal of the bottom 50% will shift the average quickly, but will also reduce the flock size to unviable levels. Selecting rams is a good compromise, as individuals contribute more to the next generation than individual ewes. Similar to selecting rams is only keeping offspring from the top 50% of the ewes. Rams may be selected both for their own traits, and this can also be based on the performance of their offspring.

more milk, or if mastitis is so widespread that the extra production potential is cancelled out by the large number of ewes with damaged udders. Equally, selecting for some traits may inadvertently select for other undesirable traits, or may select against a different desirable trait.

However, provided these limitations are borne in mind, selection for certain production traits can help produce flocks that are tailored to particular environments, management systems and producer aims. The selection process is outlined in Table 3.4.

Traits for which differences exist between breeds have proved to be amenable to selection – for example, for milk production, fecundity and wool quality. Within breed selection for sheep that are resistant (selecting for low worm egg counts) and/or resilient (selecting those which grow best in the face of high levels of challenge) to gastrointestinal roundworm infection has also been achieved.

Nutrition with Reference to Reproduction

There is no period of a ewe's life when nutrition does not have an impact on her current and future productivity. As an example, all the eggs a female mammal will ever have are generated prior to birth, while still a foetus. Restricted energy nutrition as a foetus in the uterus of an undernourished dam will reduce the potential future productivity of the ewe lamb. Failure to provide good nutrition for ewe lambs not only reduces their fertility at first mating, but also has a life-long effect on fecundity. Poor ewe lamb nutrition also restricts udder development, limiting future milk-producing capacity.

Careful nutritional management is important between weaning (when the demands of lactation cease) and mating, for the ewes achieve optimal body condition for mating (score 2.5–3.5 on a five-point scale). This helps to ensure the maintenance of good body condition throughout pregnancy, while achieving the highest ovulation rates and largest potential litter sizes. It generally takes about one month of improved nutrition to increase body condition score by 0.5 points. Ewes which are identified at weaning as being in poorer condition can be given access to better grazing than ewes which are already in better body condition. Thinner ewes can be weaned earlier, allowing them a longer period to gain body condition, while fatter ewes can be left with their lambs for a longer period. Supplementary feeding of thinner ewes can be instigated where better quality herbage is not available.

Increasing the plane of nutrition for a few weeks before mating (referred to as flushing) can result in increased ovulation rates. The effect of flushing is greatest in ewes that are in sub-optimal body condition, as they increase their food intake in response to the greater availability. Ewes that have already reached target body condition score will already be ovulating at their maximal rate and, hence, do not respond to flushing. Ewes which are in very poor condition are unlikely to respond to flushing.

The effect of flushing in ewes that are in sub-optimal body condition at mating may not be desirable, unless good nutrition can be maintained throughout pregnancy. Failure to maintain good levels of nutrition in these animals may lead to high rates of embryo loss, and increases the risk of having insufficient body stores to cope with the demands of a multiple-foetus pregnancy and rearing multiple lambs. Hence, flushing is only likely to be beneficial if ewes are in sub-optimal, but not poor, condition prior to mating, and nutritional management is such that they will have sufficient resources, in terms of body stores as well as food intake, to cope with the energy and protein demands of multiple-foetus litters.

Shorter periods of flushing can be effective where some degree of synchronisation is in place. Follicular development is controlled both by a hormone, leptin, which is affected by levels of body fat and long-term energy intake, and by glucose and insulin, which are affected by energy intake over a period of 2–3 days. Glucose and insulin elevations during the late luteal phase are sufficient to increase the numbers of follicles ovulated.

Body Condition Scoring

An objective system of body condition scoring is necessary to overcome differences in individual's perceptions of thinness and fatness, and to clearly define targets. Ewes are scored on a range of 1–5. Half scores are used to increase individual's precision, but are highly subjective, and may vary greatly, depending upon sheep breeds, wool length and operators.

The score is related to the degree of fatness in the lumbar region of the back, and is assessed in four stages:

i) The degree of prominence of the spinous processes of the lumbar vertebrae, as judged by the ease with which they can be felt and differentiated from each other.
ii) The prominence and degree of fat cover over the ends of the transverse processes, as judged by the ease with which the bones can be palpated.

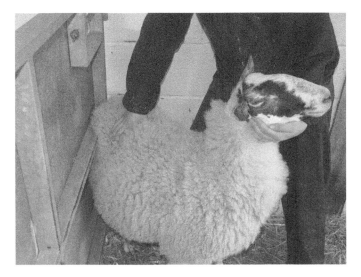

Figure 3.7 Body condition scoring by palpation of the lumbar vertebrae.

Figure 3.8 A cross-section through the lumbar spine. The numbers refer to the stages (i to iv above) in the assessment of body condition. From Russel (1984). Body condition scoring of sheep. *In Practice* **6**(3): 91–93.

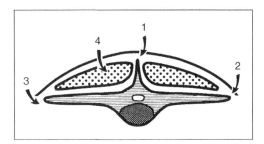

iii) The degree of muscle and fat cover beneath the transverse processes, as judged by the ease with which the fingers may be passed under these bones.

iv) The fullness of the eye muscle and fat in the angle between the spinous and transverse processes.

The process is undertaken in standing animals (Figure 3.7). These stages are shown in Figure 3.8 and described in Table 3.5.

Trace Element Deficiencies

The roles of trace element deficiencies on reducing reproductive performance are generally overstated. Copper and cobalt deficiencies cause ill thrift so may compromise the achievement of target body condition scores, with knock-on effects on reproductive performance. Iodine and selenium deficiencies have direct effects on early embryonic survival. Monitoring of the trace element status of ewes or does, and appropriate supplementation before mating, is therefore recommended. Regions in which the soil and pasture is selenium-deficient are

Table 3.5 Body condition scoring for ewes. Half scores can be allocated, but are very subjective. A score of 0 is sometimes used to describe a state of total emaciation at the point of death.

Score	Description
1	Spinous processes are prominent and sharp. Transverse processes are also sharp, the fingers pass easily under the ends and it is possible to feel between each process. Loin muscles are shallow, with no fat cover.
2	Spinous processes are prominent, but smooth. Individual processes can be felt only as fine corrugations. Transverse processes are smooth and rounded and it is possible to pass fingers under the ends with a little pressure. Loin muscles are of moderate depth, but have little fat cover.
3	Spinous processes have only a small elevation, are smooth and rounded. Individual bones can be felt only with pressure. Transverse processes are smooth and well-covered, and firm pressure is required to feel over the ends. Loin muscles are full and have a moderate degree of fat cover.
4	Spinous processes can just be detected with pressure. Ends of transverse processes cannot be felt. Loin muscles are full and have a thick covering of fat.
5	Spinous processes cannot be detected, even with firm pressure. There is a depression between the layers of fat in the position where the spinous processes would normally be felt. Transverse processes cannot be detected. Loin muscles are very full, with very thick fat cover.

generally known. Iodine-deficient soils do occur, but deficiencies are generally associated with inhibition of iodine uptake or metabolism by the thyroid gland. Feeding ewes solely on *Brassica* crops (which may contain high levels of goitrogenic substances that inhibit iodine uptake by the thyroid gland or its metabolism during mating and early pregnancy) is not recommended without provision of supplementary hay or an alternative grazing area.

Ram Nutrition

Rams must be in good body condition six weeks before introduction to the ewes, to ensure adequate sperm production and prepare them for the substantial weight loss that occurs over the mating period. A body condition of 3.5–4.0 (on a five-point scale) for the beginning of mating is desirable (Figure 3.9). Excessively fat rams, as a result of high levels of concentrate feeding, have impaired sperm production and poor libido. Rams should, therefore, be allowed to gradually recover body condition after mating, and then to maintain their target body condition score for the rest of the year. High levels of concentrate feeding of sale ram lambs should be discouraged.

Less is known about the effects of trace element deficiencies on sperm production in sheep and goats than in other species, but selenium deficiency is known to reduce sperm viability. If a trace element deficiency has been identified on farm, the rams should be supplemented in the same manner as the ewes. Excessive supplementation must be avoided.

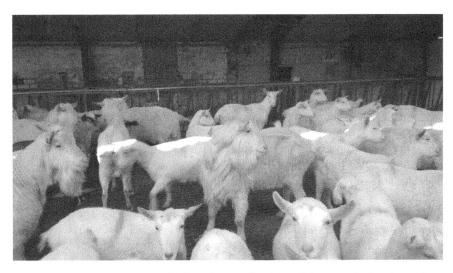

Figure 3.9 Rams and bucks must be fit and in good body condition score before the mating season, but not excessively fat. The buck in the image is suffering from ectoparasites and, hence, is likely to be sub-fertile.

Toxins

Plants such as subterranean red clover, and certain fungi which can be found on pasture, conserved forage or concentrate feed, produce compounds which mimic the female hormone oestrogen. This occasionally causes high levels of infertility in groups of ewes. Affected ewes may have swollen vulvas and a degree of udder development which is unusual for the production stage. These phytotoxins and mycotoxins, respectively, may also impair the fertility of rams.

Other plant toxins, as well as heavy metals, will interfere with reproduction, both by generalised effects on the ewes and rams, and also because embryos are particularly sensitive to toxic insult. Suspect cases should be investigated, and implicated pastures should not be grazed by ewes during the approach to mating or pregnancy.

Disease Control with Reference to the Mating Period

Various routine animal health measures are undertaken as part of a flock or herd health plan during the period between weaning and mating. Some of these treatments are required by all sheep on the farm, and some are specific for breeding ewes, rams or replacements.

Abortion Vaccination

No vaccine offers complete protection to 100% of vaccinated animals. The aim of vaccination is to produce a population where the vast majority of animals are immune, so that disease spread becomes impossible. Vaccination should be planned in advance, with careful consideration of which animals require vaccinating so as to maintain this level of immunity. Vaccination schedules differ between vaccines. Many require a primary course consisting of two injections to produce a protective level of immunity. Many also require a booster vaccination, usually annually, to keep the levels of antibodies and immune cells at protective levels.

Vaccines, especially live vaccines, are delicate products, and should be handled with care and according to the instructions on the accompanying data sheet. A commonly encountered problem is failure to keep vaccines refrigerated until the point of use. Allowing purchased vaccines to warm up, or become exposed to direct sunlight, may result in expensive failures that could be prevented by a little forethought.

Two highly effective live vaccines are currently available for the control of abortion caused by *Chlamydia abortus*. The vaccines are administered as a single intramuscular or subcutaneous injection at least four weeks prior to mating. Ewe lambs may be vaccinated from five months old. Protection lasts for at least three years, but it is common practice to vaccinate breeding ewes only once in a lifetime. These vaccines should not be used in pregnant animals, as to do so may not prevent abortions. Animals should not be under treatment with tetracycline antibiotics, as these will kill the live vaccine strain of *C. abortus* and render vaccination ineffective. *C. abortus* can cause disease in people, so appropriate care should be taken when administering the live vaccine, and pregnant women or immune compromised individuals should not handle it.

A highly effective live vaccine is available for the control of toxoplasma abortion. The vaccine is administered as a single intramuscular injection at least three weeks prior to mating. Ewe lambs may be vaccinated from five months old. The data sheet claim is for protection lasting at least two years, but vaccinating breeding ewes only once in a lifetime is generally effective, due to boosting by natural challenge. The live *Toxoplasma gondii* tachyzoite vaccine can be given on the same occasion as the chlamydial abortion vaccines. It should not be administered to pregnant ewes, as to do so may cause abortions. Toxoplasmosis is an important disease in humans, so care should be taken when administering the live vaccine, and pregnant women and immune-compromised individuals should not handle it.

An effective vaccine was promptly developed following the emergence of the Schmallenberg virus as a cause of abortions and foetal malformations in sheep. The advisability of vaccinating against Schmallenberg virus depends on local conditions and the timing of mating and pregnancy. The vaccine is administered by a single subcutaneous injection to animals from the age of 2.5 months. It should not be used in pregnant animals, and no information is available on the duration of immunity conferred.

Inactivated vaccines were developed against bluetongue virus serotype 8, following its incursion into northern Europe in 2008. The recommended administration programmes for the vaccines differ for the different products. Protective immunity lasts for six months to one year, but no booster regime has been agreed. Inactivated vaccines against serotypes other than BTV 8 are available in some countries.

Live vaccines for the control of abortion due to *Brucella melitensis* are available in some countries. These are administered either by subcutaneous injection or by application to the conjunctival lining of the eyelid. Vaccination is frequently forbidden in some countries where this disease is not endemic, including the UK.

Killed vaccines are available in Australia, New Zealand and North America for the control of abortion caused by *Campylobacter foetus foetus*. These give good protection after an initial two-dose course prior to mating. Annual boosters are required. The vaccines are unlikely to be effective for the control of abortions caused by different strains of *C. foetus foetus* in other countries.

Rift Valley fever is an important cause of abortion in small ruminants in Africa and the southern Arabian peninsula. Live, killed and mutagen-attenuated vaccines are available. Live vaccines give prolonged protection, but should not be used in pregnant animals. Killed and mutagen-attenuated vaccines are safe for use in pregnant animals.

Inactivated *Salmonella abortus ovis* vaccines are available in some countries. *Salmonella typhimurium* vaccines available in certain countries have been shown to offer cross-protection against *S. abortus ovis* abortion, as well as that directly due to *S. typhimurium*, but are ineffective in the control of abortion commonly caused by *Salmonella Montevideo* or *Salmonella Brandenburg* in the UK and New Zealand, respectively.

Lameness Control

The opportunity should be taken at weaning to assess flock lameness levels. Individual lame animals should be separated and treated. If lameness levels exceed reasonable targets of 2–5%, then the cause should be confirmed by veterinary investigation, and a control strategy developed and implemented.

Lame sheep should be treated whenever they are seen, but this vigilance should be particularly intense in the run up to mating. Lame ewes will be in poorer condition at mating, and so will have reduced fertility and fecundity. Unresolved lameness throughout pregnancy will result in thin ewes being at greater risk of pregnancy toxaemia and also being likely to rear fewer and smaller lambs (Figure 3.10). Prompt treatment within three days of detection of footrot in ewes has been shown to result in a more rapid return to soundness than delayed treatment.

Foot paring is unlikely to be necessary for the majority of sheep. Hooves generally become seriously overgrown because the animals are lame and not using the foot, and not *vice versa*. Footrot is best treated by topical application of oxytetracycline spray to the affected foot and an intramuscular injection of long-acting oxytetracycline. Paring the foot is more likely to hinder healing than to cure the problem.

Sheep Scab Control

Sheep scab, caused by the surface dwelling mange mite, *Psoroptes ovis*, is a serious threat to the health of the flock. Affected sheep are extremely pruritic (itchy), and lose body condition due to the loss of protein-rich fluid through the inflamed skin.

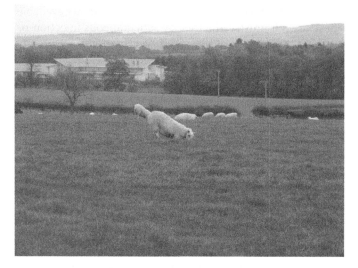

Figure 3.10 Lameness can have a profound effect on ewe reproductive performance and on the growth of their lambs.

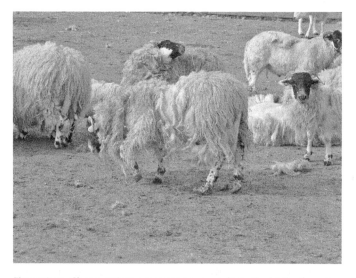

Figure 3.11 Sheep scab in pregnant ewes results in the birth of small weak lambs which impacts on lamb survival.

The impact of sheep scab on litter size, lamb birth weight and lamb growth rates can be very high (Figure 3.11). Sheep scab also has various legal implications. The disease is most frequently seen in the autumn and winter, coinciding with the mating period and early pregnancy. The movement of replacement breeding animals onto holdings can introduce disease, as can the return of sheep which have been away on summer or winter grazings.

Sheep scab control measures will depend on individual flock circumstances. These may involve:

i) maintenance of a closed flock with secure boundaries, with prompt investigation of any itchy sheep;
ii) non-closed flocks with secure boundaries and quarantine treatment of bought-in animals, or those returning from external grazings; or
iii) whole-flock treatments of non-closed flocks with unsecured boundaries, coordinated between neighbours, timed to coincide with the quarantine treatment of any bought-in animals. Treatments involve either plunge dipping in organophosphate suspensions or use of injectable macrocyclic lactone drugs.

Other External Parasite Control

Chewing lice are rarely a problem in adult ewes, and may be considered a minor nuisance in most flocks. In flocks where they are a problem, the best control measure may be the use of pour-on synthetic pyrethroids after shearing. Organophosphate plunge dips for the control of sheep scab are also effective against chewing lice. Use of synthetic pyrethroid pour-ons in long-fleeced animals will reduce numbers and help prevent itching, but it is unlikely to eliminate the louse population entirely. Underexposure of lice to lethal drug concentrations is associated with the use of pyrethroid pour-ons in long-fleeced animals selects for drug resistance. Where chewing lice have been eliminated, an effective louse treatment should be included in the quarantine procedure, to avoid their reintroduction.

Ticks often have peaks of activity in spring and in autumn. Where tick numbers are large and tick worry is a problem, then all sheep will benefit from either organophosphate plunge dipping or the use of a synthetic pyrethroid pour-on prior to high-risk periods. When naïve breeding replacements are to be introduced onto tick pastures before or during mating, then these animals may benefit from a treatment to prevent infection with tick-borne fever and louping ill, which can cause reduced sperm production in males and abortion in females. A louping ill vaccine is available.

Flystrike and fly worry tend to be less of a problem in shorn ewes than in lambs in the summer, but the risk period may extend into the autumn if temperatures permit. The need to protect ewes against flystrike and fly worry will be determined by local conditions.

Liver Fluke Control

Disease due to migrating larvae of the liver fluke, *Fasciola hepatica*, is common in the autumn (Figure 3.12). The liver damage caused by this can be severe enough to result in sudden death. Sub-acute fasciolosis can cause marked blood loss and loss of condition as well as predisposing to sudden death due to the clostridial bacterial infection, black disease.

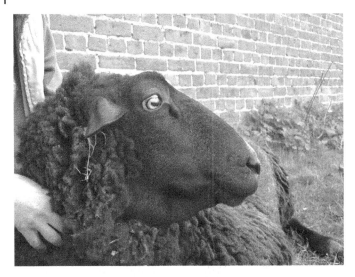

Figure 3.12 Liver fluke infection during the mating period can have profound effects on ewe reproductive performance, and can influence the survival and growth of their lambs. Note the swelling under the chin, indicative of severe hypoproteinaemia.

The liver fluke is dependent on a mud snail, *Galba truncatula*, for part of its life cycle, so higher-risk pastures can often be identified as those containing boggy areas. In wetter years, the level of fluke contamination on the pasture and the area contaminated can both rise significantly.

Mitigation of losses due to sub-acute fasciolosis can be achieved by a combination of factors. Wherever possible, grazing animals on high-risk wet pastures should be avoided during the autumn and early winter. It may be helpful to fence off specific high-risk areas. Measures aimed at reducing the mud snail habitat, such as providing hard standing areas around water troughs, planting trees and improving drainage, can be helpful.

Most sheep flocks depend upon the use of flukicidal drugs. The most versatile flukicidal drug is triclabendazole, which kills all stages of fluke larvae down to a few days after infection. On heavily contaminated pasture, sheep may need several triclabendazole treatments throughout the highest-risk period. Unfortunately, *F. hepatica* has evolved to become resistant to triclabendazole, and resistant strains are now reported in many countries. When triclabendazole resistance is present, it is necessary to use alternative flukicidal drugs, such as closantel, or nitroxynil, although these are not effective against immature stages. Hence, determining whether or not triclabendazole resistance is present is worthwhile.

Ensuring that adult fluke inside sheep, cattle or goats are killed not only has health benefits for the treated animals, but also reduces the infection challenge to the snail intermediate hosts, hence reducing the level of fluke infection of livestock during the following autumn. Animals wintered inside should be tested for fluke infection and treated, if required, before turnout. Those outwintered should be treated in the spring, depending on the disease risk assessment. All flukicides kill adult flukes, so are appropriate for this purpose. Avoiding using triclabendazole at these times reduces the selection pressure for the development of triclabednazole resistance.

Consideration should be given to avoiding the introduction of *F. hepatica*, and of resistant flukes to farms that do not already have a problem but have suitable snail habitats. In these cases, all bought-in animals should receive a quarantine treatment. Two treatments of closantel or nitroxynil, at a 6–7 week interval, are advised. Whenever possible, animals should be kept in low-risk areas such as sandy pastures, salt marshes or sheds during this period, or placed on fields being ploughed later in the year, so that any surviving resistant fluke eggs shed cannot complete their development.

Roundworm Control

Adult ewes usually have good immunity to gastrointestinal roundworms such as *Teladorsagia circumcincta* and *Trichostrongylus* spp., and do not need treating before or during the mating period. Anthelmintic treatment of ewes in the autumn may select for worms resistant to the drugs, and is unlikely to produce a significant production benefit.

The situation differs with regards to the abomasal blood-feeding roundworm, *Haemonchus contortus*. The risk of haemonchosis in ewes can be high, in particular in warmer regions following rainfall after a dry summer. Individual ewes may be affected to different levels, so selective treatments based on conjunctival colour (using the FAMACHA scoring system) may be effective and may help to reduce the risk of selection for anthelmintic resistance (Figure 3.13).

Figure 3.13 FAMACHA scores can be a useful index for the targeted selective treatment of haemonchosis in ewes.

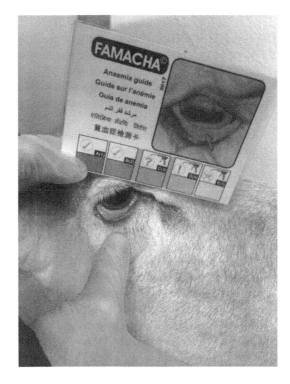

Specific Disease Control in Ewe Lambs

If ewe lambs are to be bred in their first year, they will require the same vaccinations as adults would receive on entry to the breeding flock. They will also need to have completed a primary course of any clostridial vaccination, to protect both themselves and their newborn lambs. Other routine health treatments given to the ewes should also be given to the ewe lambs.

Unlike adult sheep, ewe lambs will not have developed good immunity to gastro-intestinal roundworms, and so can suffer from parasitic gastroenteritis. An integrated control strategy of selective anthelmintic treatments and grazing management can help to ensure lack of disease and good growth rates, while exposing lambs to sufficient levels of roundworm challenge to allow the development of immunity.

Specific Disease Control in Rams

Rams do not require vaccination against agents which cause abortion only but, in some regions, it is wise to vaccinate them against diseases such as bluetongue and Rift Valley fever which cause fever, as this can affect sperm production, or against *B. melitensis*, which can infect the male genital tract and cause infertility.

Rams should receive any of the treatments given to the rest of the flock to control lameness or parasites. Unlike females, males do not develop good protective immunity against gastrointestinal roundworms, so anthelmintic treatments before mating may be helpful.

Specific Disease Control in Introduced Animals

The aim of treatments of replacement breeding sheep or goats is to bring them to the same vaccination and disease status as the rest of the flock. Where the vaccination history is unknown or suspect, introduced animals should receive the primary courses of any vaccines which are currently in use in the breeding flock. Introduced sheep should be treated for sheep scab and for chewing lice, where the home flock is louse-free.

All introduced animals should be given a quarantine treatment with a combination of different anthelmintic drug groups, such as monepantel or derquantel, and ivermectin or levamisole. They should then be turned onto contaminated grazing which has recently been grazed by the home flock, to pick up the roundworms present in the home flock and to ensure that any potentially resistant parasites which survived the quarantine treatment are a very small percentage of the total population of that species. Based on disease risk assessment, replacement animals should be treated for liver fluke, as described above.

Based on the disease risk assessment, introduced animals should be treated to remove any ticks. Potentially naïve animals introduced in the autumn to flocks in tick-affected areas should be treated with an acaracide product with persistent activity. If louping ill is known to be present, replacements should be vaccinated.

All bought-in sheep should be foot bathed twice with either 2–3% formalin or 10% zinc sulphate, to avoid the import of contagious ovine digital dermatitis or novel strains of footrot.

Mating Management

Good management during the mating period can maximise pregnancy rates, and can also aid flock management during lambing.

Length of the Mating Period

The oestrous cycle of ewes is 17 days long, and healthy adult ewes of most sheep breeds achieve 90% conception rates after natural service by a fertile ram during the breeding season. If the ewes are turned out with fertile rams for 17 days, then all should come into oestrus once during that time and be mated, with 90% becoming pregnant. If a further 17 days is allowed, then 90% of the remaining 10% should become pregnant, leaving 1% barren.

A 34-day (two oestrous cycles) mating period is considered standard for most flocks. A longer mating period can cover for deficiencies in the fertility of ewes and/or rams, but will result in a prolonged lambing period and associated problems.

Ram Numbers

Rams are expensive in terms of their value, the fact that they must be maintained all year for about one month of work, and in that the impact of an individual failure is high. Even a fit ram, with good libido and a healthy reproductive tract, can only serve a finite number of ewes in a certain time period.

Various factors must be considered when calculating the most appropriate ram-to-ewe ratio. The more synchronised the ewe flock are as to timing of oestrus, the more ewes that will need to be served on any given day. Synchrony may arise as a management decision, or as a result of the ram effect and improved nutrition on mating paddocks. Very compact lambing requires synchrony of the ewes, and so a higher ram-to-ewe ratio. Conversely, the ram-to-ewe ratio can be reduced below normal levels if a longer mating period is allowed.

Extensively managed flocks often naturally disperse into smaller sub-groups, which may be widely distributed. This limits the ability of ewes to find the ram and *vice versa*. A highly dispersed flock on very broken ground will need a higher ram-to-ewe ratio, to ensure there is always a ram within the vicinity of any oestrous ewe. Rams with larger libido and greater sperm production will succeed in serving more ewes. Ram lambs will not be able to serve as many ewes as fully mature males.

Examples of ram-to-ewe ratios appropriate to different management conditions are given in Table 3.6.

The mating group size is determined by the ram-to-ewe ratio and the number of rams to be included in a single paddock. Using a single ram with a group of ewes (single-sire mating) gives a guaranteed paternity record for any ewes mated during that period, but is a risky strategy, should the ram be unsound. Two rams may fight or, if one is far more dominant than the other, he may monopolise the ewes. However, if a ram is subfertile, the pregnancy rate will suffer. Three or more is generally considered the least risky policy.

Table 3.6 Ram : ewe ratios for different conditions.

Conditions	Appropriate ram-to-ewe ratio
Typical conditions of paddock mating lowland ewes, with a 34-day mating period and target pregnancy rate of 99%	1 : 50
Using ram lambs, or with ewes synchronised by the ram effect	1 : 20
Hormonally synchronised ewes	1 : 10
Use of superior breeding capacity rams (completely sound, high libido, scrotal circumference > 40 cm) with lowland ewes	1 : 60
If a lower pregnancy rate or a prolonged mating period is acceptable	1 : 100

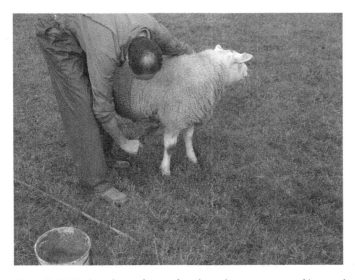

Figure 3.14 Keel marks can be used to show that rams are working, and to provide information about oestrus behaviour in ewes.

Raddle marking involves the application of paint to a ram's brisket, or the application of a harness with a crayon attached, which lies over the brisket. These mark the ewe when the ram mounts. The colour of the paint or crayon may change with ram to record paternity, or with date to allow estimation of the lambing time. Keel marks can be used to detect failure of conception by ewes returning to oestrus and being marked a second time (Figure 3.14). Non-cycling ewes are not marked.

Keel paint must be reapplied frequently, and this is most easily done if rams are trained to come to a bucket for feed. Harnesses must be well fitted or they can cause rubbing, brisket sores or injury. They should be checked regularly, and should not be used on rams with brisket sores.

Conception and Implantation

After fertilisation, the maintenance of pregnancy requires the conceptus (the result of the fusion between sperm and egg) to signal to establish pregnancy, prevent the further continuation of the oestrous cycle, and then to implant into the uterine wall. Implantation usually occurs around 14–16 days after fertilisation. During this period, the pregnancy is susceptible to stress – for example, changes in diet, or excessive moving or handling. It is recommended that minimal changes in management occur over the mating period, and for 16 days after the last ewe is mated.

Manipulation of Reproduction

It is possible to manipulate the ewes' reproductive behaviour to advance the breeding season into the transition or anoestrous periods. This can allow lambing to occur at different times of the year, in order to take advantage of economic conditions, such as higher lamb prices or reduced feed costs. It is also possible to synchronise ewes to come into oestrus within a narrow timeframe, allowing a short lambing period.

Before embarking on any reproductive manipulation programme, requisite preparation must be considered. If the breeding season is to be advanced so that a UK flock will be lambing in December, there must be sufficient shed space to house the ewes for lambing, and to keep the ewes and lambs housed until such time as the weather has improved sufficiently to allow turnout. In this example, the late pregnancy and lactation periods of greatest nutritional demand will be when there is insufficient grazing to provide the energy and protein required, so that supplementary feeding will be necessary. If synchronisation is to be used, there must be sufficient shed space or pasture allocation to allow all the ewes to be in the shed or on the lambing fields at one time. While the duration of lambing is decreased after synchronisation, the manpower required may be higher.

The Ram Effect

Exposure of ewes to the presence and smell of an adult ram can induce ewes in the transition period to begin cycling, if they have been deprived of this contact for the past month. This can advance the breeding period by 3–4 weeks in 60–70% of ewes, and cause synchronisation of 30–40% of ewes. The first oestrus is often silent, and not accompanied by oestrous behaviour. Following this silent oestrus, some ewes have a normal length cycle and some have a short cycle of 4–5 days, where the next oestrus is also silent. The first behavioural oestrus, therefore, occurs in some ewes at around 18 days after first ram introduction, and at around 24 days in the remainder.

Vasectomised rams (referred to as teasers) are often used for this purpose. They are introduced for 3–4 days, and are then removed and replaced by fertile rams about 17 days after their first introduction. One adult teaser ram per 100 ewes is generally sufficient. A higher fertile ram-to-ewe ratio is required than in the absence of the ram effect, due to the degree of synchronisation.

Photoperiod Manipulation

The trigger for ewes to begin cycling is the reduction in the photoperiod of daylight. Manipulation of the lighting period can be used to induce anoestrous ewes to cycle. Ewes need to be exposed to extended photoperiods of 15–18 hours for two months before returning to normal day length. The consequent increased hours of darkness triggers increased melatonin release, and results in a return to reproductive cyclicity. This method requires prolonged housing of sheep, and so is impractical in most settings. It becomes harder to implement at more northerly latitudes, where day length during the summer is longer.

Melatonin Implants

Increased melatonin secretion, due to increasing hours of darkness, is the signal for a resumption of cyclicity in ewes, and increased sperm production and libido in rams. This can be created artificially by the use of melatonin implants inserted subcutaneously at the base of the ear. Melatonin implants can successfully advance the breeding season into the normal period of deep anoestrus. Melatonin implants are most effective when given to both ewes and rams at the same time.

Careful planning is required, well in advance of the target date for the start of mating. Rams and ewes should be separated beyond sight, sound and smell from at least seven days before melatonin implantation. The melatonin implants should be inserted between 30–40 days before ram introduction. There is then a delay of 14–21 days before mating activity commences, with a peak of mating 25–35 days after the rams are introduced. There is no synchronisation effect with melatonin implants, but vasectomised rams can be used for the first 14 days to ensure a more compact lambing period. Conception rates to the first mating should be the same as for mating within the normal breeding period, and more than 93% of animals that do not conceive will have a second behavioural oestrus rather than returning to anoestrus.

Reproductive Hormone Manipulation

Hormone manipulation methods may be used to advance the breeding season, to synchronise oestrus, and to increase fecundity. The most appropriate method varies depending on which of these aims is most important, and on whether hormone manipulation is performed during the breeding season, during anoestrus or during the transition period.

Progesterone-releasing intravaginal sponges mimic the hormone profile of the luteal phase (the period of the oestrous cycle between ovulations). Injection of equine chorionic gonadotrophin (eCG) – also called pregnant mare's serum gonadotrophin (PMSG) – increases levels of follicle-stimulating hormone (FSH) and luteinising hormone (LH), and so causes ovulation. Sponges are placed into the ewe's vagina and left in place for 7–14 days. The sponge is then removed, and PMSG is administered to advance and synchronise the breeding season.

4

Husbandry and Health Planning to Prepare for Lambing: Nutritional Management of Pregnant Ewes and Does

The nutritional requirements of ewes and does vary greatly throughout pregnancy and lactation. In the first two-thirds of pregnancy, the energy and protein demands are only slightly higher than those of maintenance of the ewe. The energy and protein requirements increase substantially in the last third of pregnancy as a consequence of growth of the foetuses and other products of conception. Adequate nutrition throughout pregnancy is important, to ensure that conceived embryos survive through to birth and that ewes are in optimal body condition for lambing, to avoid ewe and lamb losses as a result of metabolic and nutritional diseases and to allow satisfactory milk production and lamb growth rates to weaning.

Nutritional management impacts economically upon the lambing percentage, ewe mortality rates, lamb survival, lamb growth rates and flock replacement rates.

Early and Mid-pregnancy

Early pregnancy is the period when the embryo develops the major organ systems. A concern at this stage is to avoid the ingestion of substances that could damage the developing embryo. Improved pastures are generally unlikely to contain harmful plants, and extensively managed animals are unlikely to graze harmful plants unless little else is available. Overdosing with anthelmintic drugs should be avoided, as this can cause foetal deformities.

The aim during early pregnancy should be to maintain the body condition score of ewes that were at, or below, target for mating. Fat ewes (score 4.0–5.0 on a five-point scale) can afford to lose up to 9% of their body weight (about 0.75 units of body condition score) during this period, and should do so to reduce the risks in later pregnancy of vaginal prolapse, pregnancy toxaemia and dystocia.

During mid-pregnancy, the placenta undergoes the majority of its growth. The additional nutritional demands for placental development are low but, nevertheless, severe nutritional restriction at this time should be avoided. The foetus is reliant on its placenta for oxygen and nutrients, so an underdeveloped placenta will restrict foetal growth. Ewes with chronic disease problems, or those which underwent severe malnutrition before and during mid-pregnancy, may give birth to stunted lambs as a result. Ewe lambs which are overfed during mid-pregnancy

Practical Lambing and Lamb Care – A Veterinary Guide, Fourth Edition.
Neil Sargison, James Patrick Crilly and Andrew Hopker.
© 2018 John Wiley & Sons Ltd. Published 2018 by John Wiley & Sons Ltd.

divert energy to their own growth rather than pregnancy. The placenta which develops is consequently smaller than it would otherwise be, resulting in growth-retarded lambs.

Nutritional stress during mid-pregnancy needs to be severe and prolonged before it affects the lambing percentage. Ewes which were at, or above, target body condition score for mating can afford to lose up to 9% of their body weight during this period.

Late Pregnancy Energy Nutrition

The energy requirements of ewes increase dramatically in the final eight weeks of pregnancy. The energy demands of ewes carrying multiple foetuses often cannot be met from their diet alone and, hence, it is normal for them to mobilise body fat and glycogen reserves during this period.

Ewes above a condition score of 2.5 (on a five-point scale) a month before lambing can lose 0.5 units of condition score in the approach to lambing without adverse effects. Body condition loss at this rate provides the equivalent of 2 MJ of metabolisable energy per day, which reduces the required energy density of the diet. Thin ewes (score 1.0–2.0 on a five-point scale) cannot afford to mobilise further body reserves, so must be fed more than those ewes that have maintained target body condition scores.

These nutritional requirements generally necessitate the feeding of a more energy-dense ration during late pregnancy. While this can be achieved in non-pastoral systems using high quality silage alone, supplementary concentrate feeding is necessary in most cases. There is, however, a limit on how much concentrate can be fed without resulting in acidification of the forestomach, with a resultant decrease in the efficacy of digestion.

As a rule, concentrates should never constitute more than 60% of the dry matter intake of a sheep. For an average 70–80 kg lowland ewe, no more than 0.5 kg of grain, by-product or compounded concentrates should be given in a single feed. All changes in diet should be gradual, to avoid disturbances to rumen function. It is preferable, wherever possible, for the maximum amount of energy in the diet to be derived from forage. This is not only better for the ewe's digestive function, but is also economically the most cost-effective.

Forage analysis enables the energy deficit from feeding hay or silage alone to be calculated, and the diet then adjusted to include sufficient concentrate feed to meet the ewes' requirements. Where analysis of feeds is not available, standard figures may be used instead, although these cannot truly reflect what is being included in the ration.

While not identical to sheep, the requirements and dry matter intakes of goats during gestation are very similar. Goats have a reputation for being able to perform better when fed poorer quality forage than either cattle or sheep. This may reflect more the fact that goats are extremely selective feeders and seek out the best quality parts of poorer quality forage. Ideally, forage should be available *ad lib*, and 15–20% discarded may be expected.

The traditional approach to concentrate feeding is to increase the amount of concentrate in a stepwise fashion, to keep pace with the increasing energy demands of the pregnancy. When concentrate feeding is started depends on the energy provision from the forage and the body condition of the ewes. In most cases, feeding of twins and triplets begins 8–6 weeks before lambing, and that of singles about four weeks before lambing.

An alternative approach involves flat rate concentrate feeding, beginning about 10–8 weeks before the lambing. This involves feeding a diet which provides in excess of energy requirements at first. This is stored in body reserves and is mobilised later, when the diet provides insufficient energy. An advantage of this system is that the levels of concentrate feeding at any one time are lower than during the later stages of a stepwise feeding regime, so that the risk of ruminal acidosis, impairing the efficiency of digestion and maximal utilisation of forage, is reduced.

Root crops such as turnips, swedes and fodder beet are relatively energy-dense and may be considered as wet concentrates in terms of energy provision. Unlike cereal and by-product based concentrates, their capacity to cause ruminal acidosis is limited, and they may form up to 90% of the diet by dry matter weight. However, a very large fresh weight must be fed, due to the low dry matter content of these foods. Root crops are often fed directly, or are harvested and then left on the field surface for sheep to consume. If sheep are fed on root crops, they must have access to some hay, silage or grass, due to the low fibre content of the former. Root crops are also very low in protein, so some form of protein supplementation will be required.

Leafy *Brassica* crops are a good and economic energy source, but contain factors which can lead to anaemia, or may reduce the availability of iodine from the diet if fed for prolonged periods. A grass area is required, or hay or silage should be provided. If late pregnant ewes are run on *Brassica* crops, judicious iodine supplementation may be required in order to prevent iodine deficiency in the lambs.

Ewes lambing outdoors, or those at pasture until the very last weeks of pregnancy, will receive some of their energy intake from grazed herbage. How much energy this can provide will depend on the quality and amount of grazing available. Energy provision is greatest from new grass leys containing species such as Italian ryegrass. Older meadows or mixed-species grassland may not meet the levels of production of these leys, but may provide more protein and be productive under more challenging growing conditions. Growing grass is more energy- and protein-dense than flowering grass and dead, standing grass. Spring grass tends to be more energy- and protein-dense than autumn growth. The dry matter provision per hectare can be calculated on the basis of sward height and supplementation provided.

Grass grown in relatively cool, moist conditions, such as those that prevail in north-west Europe and New Zealand, tends to have higher nutritional value than grasses that grow in warmer areas. The daily grass growth in the tropics can be many times greater than in temperate climates, provided that sufficient water is available, due to the higher temperatures. However, the digestibility of the grass tends to be lower, as are sugar and protein levels. Care should be taken, therefore, in extrapolating feeding guidelines from higher latitudes to the tropics.

Protein Intakes in Late Pregnancy

While energy is important for foetal growth, protein is also required. Sufficient protein intake is necessary for efficient forestomach digestion, and for optimal quality and quantity of colostrum and milk production. Higher levels of dietary protein provision have been associated with significantly lower worm egg outputs from ewes in the periparturient period, presumably related to better immune function.

Whether or not supplementary protein is required depends on the basis of the diet. Growing spring grass is often protein-rich, while root crops and straw are low in protein, and hay and silage may be very varied. Protein supplementation might include provision of legumes as crushed seeds (soya, beans, or peas) or as forage (alfalfa, grass silage containing peas, high clover pastures). Many commercial compound rations are formulated to contain a certain level of protein. The crude protein content of compound rations is shown on their label (for example, 18% CP), but the quality of the protein, and the relative levels of effective rumen degradable protein (ERDP) and digestible undegraded protein (DUP), are also important.

Where high-quality silage is available and meets the energy requirements of the majority of ewes, then protein supplementation is all that is required. For example, with 11 MJ ME/ kg DM silage feeding, supplementary feeding of soya for the last three weeks of pregnancy, at a rate of 100 g per lamb carried, is sufficient.

Mineral and Trace Element Nutrition

The major minerals include sodium, potassium, calcium, magnesium and phosphorus (in the form of phosphate). Deficiencies of potassium are rarely seen, as most plant material is relatively rich in potassium. The sodium-to-potassium ratio of spring grass and maize silage is very low, and this can lead to problems of magnesium metabolism. Hypocalcaemia is usually seen pre-lambing, and is often triggered by stressful episodes. Absolute deficiencies are rare and many problems relate to a failure of mobilisation from the skeletal store. These problems may be compounded in animals which are housed for long periods, due to vitamin D deficiency. Magnesium levels are usually adequate in most diets, but may be low if the animals are on a straw-based diet which is supplemented by straights, rather than commercially compounded concentrates. Phosphate intakes are impaired in cases of severe gastrointestinal parasitism. While phosphorus deficiency is rare in temperate areas, the very low phosphate content of the diet of sheep and goats grazing on tropical and subtropical rangelands can result in deficiencies. This manifests as poor growth rates and a tendency to chew bones they might encounter – referred to as 'pica'.

Female goats which are mated at too young an age, or too small a size, may develop angular limb deformities during pregnancy when the combined calcium demands of maternal and foetal skeletal growth outstrip supply.

Copper, selenium, cobalt and iodine trace elements are vital for sheep health. Low copper levels result in failure of development of parts of the central nervous system of lambs, causing a disease known as swayback. Care must be taken with supplementation, as sheep are very prone to copper toxicity. Certain breeds are more effective at extracting copper from the diet than others, and so are more prone to copper toxicity. Feeds containing high, but unknown, levels of copper should not be fed to sheep. Cattle and pig feeds contain higher levels of copper than sheep can tolerate, and should never be fed to sheep. Adult goats have a higher tolerance of copper than do sheep, but kids appear to be as sensitive as lambs to copper toxicity.

Low selenium and/or vitamin E levels result in a failure of the body to deal with free radical by-products of respiration. Free radicals damage cell membranes and contents. Free radical production is especially high in energetically active tissues, like the heart and postural muscles, so the first observed clinical signs of deficiency relate to heart failure and muscular exhaustion in neonatal lambs. Where selenium deficiency is known to be a problem, ewes should be supplemented in late pregnancy to avoid white muscle disease in lambs. Vitamin E is abundant in fresh green leaves, so most sheep are at low risk of deficiency, with the exception of those on straw and concentrate diets.

In arid or semi-arid areas with alkaline soils (for example, in parts of the western USA), soil selenium concentrations can be relatively high. Certain plants concentrate selenium within their foliage, so animals grazing these can develop selenium toxicity. This manifests as poor growth, hair loss, hoof splitting and shedding, weakness, pulmonary oedema and necrosis of various muscles, including the heart.

The effect of low cobalt on pregnant ewes and neonatal lambs is less marked than in growing lambs, but severe deficiency has been loosely associated with poorer milk and colostrum production, and reduced lamb survival.

Primary iodine deficiencies are mostly confined to inland and mountainous areas. Secondary iodine deficiency more frequently seen and is related to the ingestion of goitrogenic substances in a variety of forage crops, including grass, clover and brassicae. These substances interfere with the uptake of iodine by the thyroid gland, or production of iodine-containing hormones. Iodine-deficient ewes may give birth to stillborn or weak lambs. In extreme cases, lambs are born with distended abdomens, a sparse wool coat and greatly enlarged thyroid glands. Others are born with less obvious thyroid gland enlargement, but are susceptible to hypothermia.

Zinc deficiency is occasionally seen in goats. At least one hereditary zinc absorption or utilisation disorder has been suggested, with zinc deficiency seen in some individuals, even when dietary levels appear to be normal and other goats in the herd unaffected. Clinical signs of zinc deficiency include an abnormal retention of the surface layer of skin cells, leading to a scurfy appearance (parakeratosis), joint stiffness, excessive salivation and reduced testicular size and libido.

Measuring Nutritional Adequacy in Late Pregnancy

There is generally a good level of understanding of the protein and energy requirements of pregnant ewes, the nutrient composition of forage and concentrate feeds, and the principles of ration formulation. However, the nutritional requirements of individual ewes are not standard, and the nutrient composition and availability of different batches of forage and concentrate feeds varies. It is, therefore, necessary first to adopt a prescribed nutritional management strategy, based on ration formulation and experience, and then to monitor its adequacy at strategic times by body condition scoring and measurement of metabolite concentrations in blood samples.

Body Condition Scoring

The simplest measure of energy intake is body condition, although this only provides only historical information. Regular body condition scoring, before and throughout pregnancy, allows for the ration to be modified whenever targets are not met. Identifying unexpectedly low condition scores can indicate a disease problem and can allow for pre-emptive planning.

Goats and some breeds of sheep tend to store the majority of their body fat reserves in the omentum and around the kidneys, so the lumbar region, which is used for condition scoring in sheep, is far less reliable in goats. It is recommended that the sternal region, as well as the lumbar region, should be palpated in goats.

Ration Analysis

It can sometimes be a useful exercise to work out whether or not the diet makes sense on paper. This requires information about forage and concentrate analysis and ewe body weights. Information about forage dry matter (DM) and metabolisable energy (ME) is helpful, but standard figures can be used if this information is not available.

Ewe dry matter intake (DMI) in late pregnancy is 2.1% of bodyweight. If the ewe is fed forage alone, the energy provision can be calculated. For example, for a 70 kg ewe being fed good quality silage (11 MJ ME/kg DM):

$$\text{Energy provided by forage} = (0.021 \text{ BW } (\text{kg})) \times \text{ME of silage}$$
$$= (0.021 \times 70) \times 11 = 16.17 \text{ MJ ME per day.}$$

The energy provision of the diet with the concentrate feed present can then be calculated. Feeding concentrate usually results in the ewes preferentially eating the concentrate first, with DMIs of forage falling as a result (the total amount of DM consumed does not change), and this assumption is used in the ration-checking calculations (exceptions to this rule include when ewes are fed a straw-based diet, where the inclusion of concentrate increases the DMI overall as it increases the rate of digestion in the rumen).

The energy provided from the concentrate is calculated from the amount fed (kg) × DM percentage × ME content. For example, for a 70 kg ewe being fed 0.4 kg of an 86% DM, 12.5 MJ ME/kg DM concentrate per day, and with good quality silage (11 MJ ME/kg DM):

Energy provided by concentrate $= 0.4 \times 0.86 \times 12.5 = 4.3$ MJ.

In this example, feeding both forage and concentrates

Energy provided by forage $= \big((0.021 \times 70) - (0.4 \times 0.86) \big) \times 11 = 12.4$ MJ.

Hence, the total energy provided by the ration $= 12.4 + 4.3 = 16.7$ MJ ME per day.

Calculating the protein provision is more difficult, as the protein available to the ewe consists of that which is not broken down in the rumen but is digested in the small intestine (DUP), and the protein produced by the microbial digestion and both protein and non-protein nitrogen sources in the forestomach, which are then digested in the small intestine as microbial crude protein (MCP). MCP production is limited by either fermentable metabolisable energy (FME) provision or nitrogen availability (ERDP), whichever is smaller.

Let us take the same example of a 70 kg ewe being fed good quality (11 MJ ME/kg, 18% CP, 25% DM) silage only. For grass silage with an ME of 11 MJ/kg, the FME would be approximately 9 MJ/kg.

The daily DMI $= 0.021 \times 70 = 1.47$ kg, so the daily FME intake $= 1.47 \times 9 = 13.23$ MJ FME. For grass silage with 18% CP at moderate ruminal outflow rates, the ERDP is 14.9% and the DUP 2.6%.

The daily DUP intake $= 1.47 \times 0.026 = 0.038$ kg (38 g).

It is necessary to determine if ERDP is limiting on MCP production.

Daily ERDP (g) required $=$ FME $(MJ) \times 10 = 13.23$ MJ $\times 10 = 132.3 \, g$.

Daily ERDP provided $= 1.47 \times 0.149 = 0.219$ kg $(219 \, g)$.

Hence, in this example, ERDP is not limiting and, thus, the limit on MCP production is FME. When ERDP is not limiting:

MCP $=$ FME $\times 10 \times 0.635 = 132.3 \times 0.635 = 84$ g (0.635 is the conversion efficacy of energy to MCP in the presence of sufficient ERDP).

Thus, total protein provision is MCP + DUP $= 84 + 38 = 122$ g.

It can be seen from this example that the limit on the amount of protein the ewe can acquire from top-quality silage is the energy provision, as good-quality grass silage is rich in ERDP. The protein density of the diet could be increased by increasing energy provision, perhaps by providing a small amount of barley or molasses and thereby increasing FME availability, but this will substitute for grass silage and may end up dropping the protein density if too much is provided. The alternative approach is to provide a small amount of a very DUP rich supplement, such as soya.

Metabolic Profiling

Metabolic profiling involves blood sampling of a representative sample of each management group of ewes and measuring the levels of various parameters. The levels of these give some information on the metabolic state of the animal.

Elevated levels of beta-hydroxybutyrate (BOHB) indicate that the ewe is mobilising body energy stores. For individual ewes, levels above 1.1 mmol/l represent inadequacy of energy nutrition. For groups of animals fed according to litter size, body condition and predicted lambing date a mean value of 1.0 mmol/l is used, while a mean value of 0.8 mmol/l is used for mixed groups. Whenever these targets are exceeded, it is possible to refer to standard reference curves for the weight of ewe in order to estimate the dietary energy deficiency (the reference curves were published by Angus Russel (1985): Nutrition of the pregnant ewe. *In Practice* 7(1): 23–28.)

Low levels of blood urea N (BUN) indicate insufficient levels of effective rumen-degradable protein (ERDP) in the ration being fed at the time of sampling. Low levels of ERDP limit the activity of forestomach microbes, which severely limits the protein available to the ewe. Blood urea levels should be above 2.0 mmol/l.

Albumin concentrations reflect longer-term protein intake, but low levels may also indicate chronic disease, especially liver fluke or *Haemonchus contortus* infection. Target low albumin levels tend to fall from about 30 g/l at six weeks before lambing, to about 26 g/l at lambing. Precise target are set by the diagnostic laboratories, and also depend on whether serum or plasma is analysed.

Magnesium values tend to vary with feed intakes. Variable magnesium values across the group suggest that some animals feed intakes are insufficient. Low values across the group may reflect low dietary magnesium content, but may also reflect a low sodium : potassium ratio. Plasma magnesium concentrations should be above 0.7 mmol/l.

The optimal time to sample pregnant ewes is 3–4 weeks before the start of lambing. If sampled too soon, the ewes may not yet be under much metabolic demand from pregnancy. However, if sampling is too late, the opportunity to make changes to the diet is limited.

Inspection of Foodstuffs and Feeding

The theory of ration formulation must be supported by common sense observation of feeding behaviour, and of the manner in which the feed is presented.

Sheep and goats have a dominance hierarchy, sometimes allowing some animals to monopolise the feed space and to prevent subordinate animals from feeding. Some animals may be content with the food they have, while others are always looking for more or better food. These considerations may be compounded when feeding space is limited.

Forage should always be available, and feed spaces should never be empty or inaccessible (Figure 4.1). Daily inspection is required. When concentrates are fed, they should be spread evenly throughout the feed space (Figure 4.2). A minimum feed space of 15 cm for *ad lib* forage provision and 45 cm for limited concentrate feed provision is recommended, but these figures should be increased for large sheep, ewes with multiple foetuses, and horned sheep.

Spoiled feed is unpalatable, has much reduced nutritional properties, and will dissuade animals from eating in contact good feed. It can also be a risk to sheep

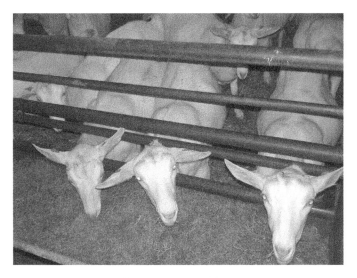

Figure 4.1 Forage should always be available.

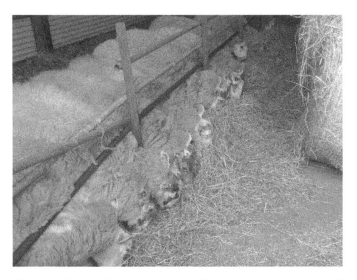

Figure 4.2 Enough feeding space should be provided to ensure that all ewes in a group have access to concentrate feed at the same time. Here, the concentrates are being fed on top of the forage.

health, causing problems such as fungal abortion or listeriosis. Uneaten feed should be cleared away regularly. Forage with holes in it suggests that the food on offer is largely not to the liking of the sheep, and that they are searching through it for more palatable segments (Figure 4.3).

Clean, fresh water should always be provided. While intake of water from troughs by sheep on pasture in the winter is minimal, housed late-pregnant ewes fed on drier diets will drink substantial amounts – up to eight litres per ewe per day. Restricted water provision will restrict feed intakes. At least 1.5 cm per ewe

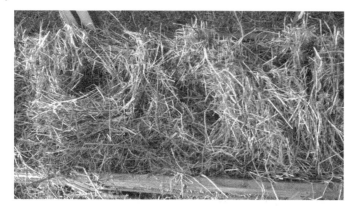

Figure 4.3 Spoiled forage should be removed daily to avoid wastage through selective feeding, as shown by the holes that have been made into this silage bunker.

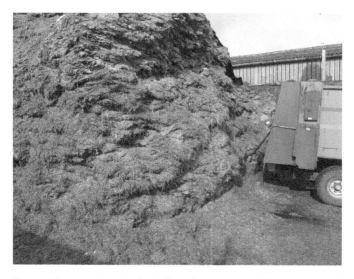

Figure 4.4 A poorly maintained silage face causes spoilage, reducing the nutritive value of the forage and increasing the risk of multiplication of harmful bacteria.

water trough space is required. The water pressure should be sufficient to keep the trough full. Sheep standing to wait for water should be avoided.

Forage should be stored in such a way that minimises spoilage (Figure 4.4). Hay and straw should be kept dry. Mouldy hay and straw should not be fed to pregnant ewes. Hay and straw contaminated with cat faeces is a major risk for *Toxoplasma* abortion, and should not be fed to pregnant ewes. Silage clamp management should aim to keep a smooth, compact face, minimising spoilage doe to ingress of air (Figure 4.5). Big bale silage should be well compacted, and the bales should not be deformed. The wrapping should be intact, otherwise the introduction of air will allow spoilage.

Hard feed should be stored in a clean, dry container which excludes vermin, birds and cats (Figure 4.6). Mouldy feed should be discarded.

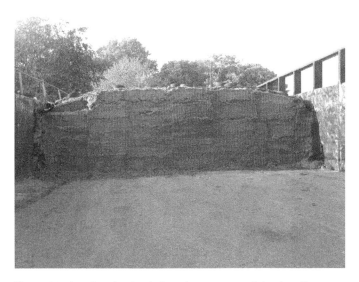

Figure 4.5 A well-maintained silage face ensures minimal spoilage.

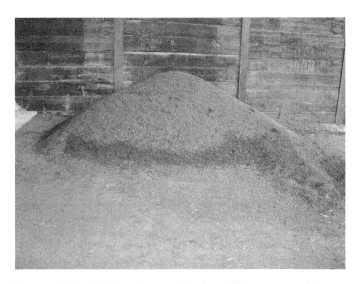

Figure 4.6 Hard feed must be stored in dry and biosecure conditions to avoid spoilage and contamination with harmful pathogens.

Insufficient lying space per ewe will limit rumination activity, and so reduce feed intakes and digestion efficacy (Figure 4.7). At least $1.8\,\text{m}^2$ should be available for every pregnant ewe.

Toxic Plants

Various plants that are embryotoxic, or otherwise interfere with pregnancy, are shown in Table 4.1.

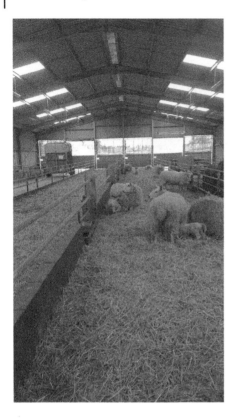

Figure 4.7 A comfortable environment is important to ensure good digestion and feed intake.

Table 4.1 Potentially embryotoxic plants (plants which are generally toxic to sheep are not included).

Plant	Problem
Veratrum spp. (false hellebores)	Foetal deformities. Around day 14 of pregnancy, consumption results in cyclopia and facial deformities. Consumption around day 25 causes limb deformities.
Gutierrezia spp. (snakeweed)	Embryonic death and low birth weight.
Tobacco plants.	Foetal neuromuscular inhibition.
Sorghum spp. (fodder grass)	Foetal dysplasias and low birth weights.
Trachymene spp. (lace flower)	Forelimb deformities.
Brassica spp.	Goitre, low birth weight, poor coat quality, low vigour and poor viability.
Astragalus spp. (locoweed)	Interferes with progesterone production and can lead to abortion.
Lupinus spp. (lupins)	Interferes with progesterone production and can lead to abortion.

Feeding Ewes in Extensive Systems

In extensive systems, such as hefted hill flocks in the UK, or flocks on range-lands in the USA or Australia, provision of supplementary feed is often diffi-cult or impossible. Estimating the dietary provision is difficult, due to the diverse nature of vegetation on these grazings, and the selective feeding of sheep and goats. The main nutritional aims are to ensure that any trace ele-ment deficiencies are corrected, to move thin ewes and those scanned with multiple foetuses to any improved grazing which is available, and to ensure that the metabolic drain of disease is minimised. Regular body condition scor-ing, along with prior experience, is used to determine if the carrying capacity of the land is being exceeded. This varies from season to season and from year to year.

Ultrasound Scanning

Ultrasound scanning for pregnancy is usually performed between days 45 and 90 of pregnancy. This is usually performed using a sector scanner with a rotating transducer, applied to the ewes' abdomen on the wool-free region just in front of the udder. Pregnancy is recognised by the presence of anechoic fluid within the uterus. In late pregnancy, the foetus may be so large as to fill the screen, which can make interpretation of foetal numbers difficult. In early pregnancy, before the development of the cotyledons – which may appear C-shaped or O-shaped, depending on the plane of view– pregnancy can only be confirmed by the detec-tion of the embryo.

There are various benefits to ultrasound scanning of ewes. It can detect a fertil-ity or abortion problem early, allowing investigation and potential control meas-ures to be put in place rapidly. Barren ewes can be detected early, and then sold when prices are high, avoiding the cost of feeding non-productive animals. Determination of foetal numbers allows management of ewes appropriate to their energy requirements (Figure 4.8), and also allows early planning for artifi-cial rearing of lambs if the percentage of multiple pregnancies is higher than expected. If the percentage of single pregnancies is higher than expected, it allows early instigation of the problem.

It is possible to determine foetal age from certain measurements, such as abdominal diameter and head width. This can allow estimated lambing dates to be given, and may highlight infertile rams if the dates of entry and removal to groups of ewes are known.

Scanning of goats has the same benefits as for sheep, with the additional advantage of the detection and treatment of hydrometra. Hydrometra is a false pregnancy, occurring when the corpus luteum persists in the absence of an embryo. Fluid accumulates within the uterus, so the animal appears pregnant. When the corpus luteum regresses, the false pregnancy ends and the fluid is expelled. Risk factors for the occurrence of hydrometra include out-of-season

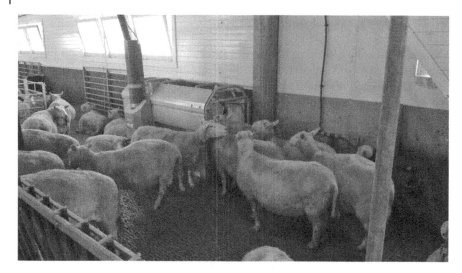

Figure 4.8 Results of ultrasound scanning for foetal numbers should be used to ensure precise nutritional management of pregnant ewes. These ewes are fed concentrates in accordance with their litter size, body condition and expected lambing date.

breeding, delayed breeding during the breeding season, treatment with eCG, phytoestrogens in the diet and causes of early embryonic death, such as border disease or toxoplasmosis. Treatment involves giving luteolytic drugs (5–10 mg of PGF2a or 125–150 µg of cloprostenol) to lyse the corpus luteum.

5

Husbandry and Health Planning to Prepare for Lambing: Health Management of Pregnant Ewes and Does

Control of Endemic Diseases

Vaccination

Vaccination boosters given to ewes during late pregnancy raise levels of antibodies in colostrum, protecting lambs against specific diseases. Comprehensive clostridial disease vaccination programmes are needed to protect lambs against the enterotoxaemias, lamb dysentery and pulpy kidney, and tetanus in particular. The data sheet of the individual vaccine used should be consulted for the recommended timing of the primary and booster doses boosters. Vaccination also provides some protection of the ewe from gangrenous conditions caused by other clostridial bacteria, which affect the reproductive tract following damage at lambing.

Some multicomponent clostridial vaccines also include pneumonia-causing bacteria, and so offer a short period of protection of the lambs from disease caused by *Mannheimiahaemolytica* and *Bibersteiniatrehalosi*.

Boosters of other vaccines may be timed for this period if passive transfer of immunity to lambs is required. Examples include louping ill vaccine.

The data sheet should be consulted prior to administration of vaccines to pregnant ewes. Certain products, such as footrot vaccines, should not be given prior to lambing.

Ewes are sometimes vaccinated against orf prior to lambing. While this helps to protect the ewes, it is less effective in protecting the lambs than vaccinating the young lambs themselves.

Goats, like sheep, should be vaccinated against clostridial disease prior to kidding. However, no clostridial vaccines are licensed for goats in the UK, and the duration of immunity that develops following vaccination with sheep vaccines is limited. It is, therefore, recommended that goats be vaccinated three to four times a year with a clostridial vaccine. The immune response to the vaccine appears to be greatest when the number of different clostridial strains included is lowest so, in the absence of a specific herd problem, it is generally recommended that a vaccine which covers only *C. perfringens* and *C. tetani* is given.

Practical Lambing and Lamb Care – A Veterinary Guide, Fourth Edition.
Neil Sargison, James Patrick Crilly and Andrew Hopker.
© 2018 John Wiley & Sons Ltd. Published 2018 by John Wiley & Sons Ltd.

Liver Fluke Control

Ewes grazing high-risk wet fields during the autumn and winter may acquire a fluke burden. These animals may benefit from treatment after housing, or before lambing, with a flukicidal drug. Testing groups of ewes to establish whether they are infected by submission of faeces for microscopic examination for fluke eggs can allow treatments to be targeted towards those animals that might benefit from removal of the extra metabolic demands of fluke infection.

Sheep Scab Control

Sheep scab can cause extreme pruritus and significant protein loss through the inflamed skin. This can have profound effects on lamb birth weights and the milk production of ewes, with consequent high lamb mortality rates. Itchy sheep should be investigated, so that appropriate treatment can be instigated well before the start of lambing. Heavily pregnant sheep should not be plunge dipped.

Control of Gastrointestinal Roundworms

Ewes' immunity to gastrointestinal roundworms is relaxed during the last few weeks of pregnancy and throughout the first 6–8 weeks of lactation, resulting in a periparturient rise in their faecal egg output. As lactation ceases, ewes recover their immunity, and worm numbers and faecal egg outputs tend to return to pre-lambing levels.

Dosing of ewes at turnout to pasture is common practice, with the objective of controlling pasture contamination from the periparturient rise in egg output. However, with the emergence of anthelmintic resistance, worm control strategies that rely on anthelmintic drugs have become ineffective and need to be questioned. The periparturient rise in egg output is less marked in single-bearing ewes than in multiple-bearing ewes, and can be reduced by dietary protein supplementation.

The timing of dosing and linked choice of wormer are important. Ewes are likely to become re-infected quickly if they are still experiencing a relaxation of immunity and, on contaminated pasture, when treatment with a conventional non-persistent anthelmintic drug ceases. Selection for anthelmintic resistance is minimal under these conditions, albeit the benefit of treatment, in terms of subsequent pasture contamination, is also low. Consequently, repeated or long-acting or persistent anthelmintic treatments have been advocated, with the aim of reducing pasture infectivity for the lambs later in the season. However, this can be highly selective for anthelmintic resistant worms, because there may be a prolonged period during which any resistant survivors of treatment are not diluted by susceptible worms on pasture.

A compromise must, therefore, be reached between reduction in pasture larval contamination for the subsequent grazing lambs, and avoiding high selection pressure for anthelmintic resistance. This may involve leaving a proportion of ewes untreated, or treating early in the post-lambing phase to ensure that ewes become re-infected with unselected parasites before their immunity is fully restored. There are also no hard and fast guidelines as to how many ewes to leave untreated, nor how long to delay after lambing before treatment. These factors need to be considered as part of a veterinary health plan, then monitored and adjusted accordingly.

Similar principles apply to goats, although the manner in which they do not develop good immunity to gastrointestinal worms means that control of pasture larval contamination levels is more difficult.

Abortion

Identifying an Abortion Problem

A certain number of abortions will occur in any given flock of sheep. Although this may relate to individual disease problems of the ewe, it is of little concern when it comes to the flock as a whole. In any flock, multiple ewes aborting during a short period of time is a cause for concern, and should prompt further investigation. An overall abortion rate of 2% is considered to be within normal limits. Higher rates or abortions, accompanied by ewe deaths, are indications for further investigation.

Abortion occurring in housed ewes in late pregnancy is usually obvious (Figure 5.1). However, abortion in early or mid-pregnancy or in extensively managed outdoor-lambing flocks may be harder to detect. Resorbing foetuses are sometimes identified at the time of ultrasound scanning for pregnancy. Large numbers of ewes found not to be in lamb at the end of lambing should also prompt investigation.

The most common causes of abortion in UK sheep flocks are chlamydial abortion, toxoplasmosis, salmonellosis and campylobacteriosis. However, other

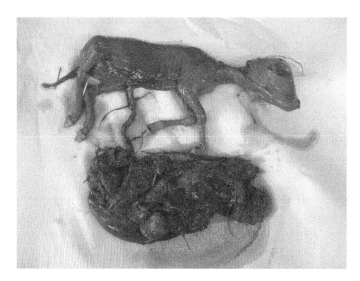

Figure 5.1 A mummified aborted foetus. Ewe abortion is always a harrowing experience.

Table 5.1 Abortion in UK sheep.

Cause of abortion	Clinical signs	Source of infection	Zoonotic potential
Toxoplasma gondii (toxoplasmosis)	High barren rates, abortion at any stage of pregnancy. Stillbirths, mummified lambs, weak lambs.	Infected cats	Yes
Chlamydia abortus (enzootic abortion)	Abortion in the last third of pregnancy. Stillbirths and weak lambs.	Carrier aborting or previously aborted ewes	Yes
Salmonella Montevideo and other salmonella spp	Abortion in the second half of pregnancy. Autolysed lambs and sick ewes. Ewe deaths.	Carrier ewes or wildlife	Yes
Campylobacter foetus foetus	Abortion in the last third of pregnancy.	Introduced with carrier ewes or spread by birds	No
Broder disease virus	High barren rates, abortions and birth of fine-boned, hairy shaker lambs. High incidence of neonatal disease.	Introduced with persistently infected sheep	No
Listeriosis	Late abortions and septicaemia.	Poor silage	Yes
Anaplasmaphagocytophilium (Tick borne fever)	High barren rates. Abortion. Increased incidence of other diseases.	*Ixodesricinus* ticks	Yes
Coxiellaburnettii (Q fever)	Abortion and birth of weak lambs.	Aerosol spread from aborted material, urine, faeces or milk. Potential tick transmission	Yes
Schmallenberg virus	Birth or deformed lambs.	Infected *Culicoides* midges	No
Fungi or mycotoxins	Abortion at any stage.	Mouldy feed	No
Campylobacter jejuni	Abortion in late pregnancy and diarrhoea.	Many species can act as carriers. Birds are often implicated	Yes
Other bacteria	Abortion at any stage.	Various	Yes

causes are important in affected flocks. The features of causes of abortion are described in Table 5.1.

Various other diseases causing abortion in sheep around the world are shown in Table 5.2. The risk of introduction of these diseases to new countries cannot be overlooked.

Table 5.2 Other diseases causing abortion around the world.

Cause of abortion	
Anaplasmosis	*Anaplasmaosis* is spread by ticks. The protozoal parasite invades red blood cells, causing an immune-mediated extravascular haemolytic anaemia. Abortion may occur. Control is by control of ticks.
Bluetongue virus	Bluetongue virus is spread by biting midges. It is seen in Africa, Asia and Europe. Clinical signs include high fever, oedema of the muzzle and tongue, swelling of the coronary band and abortion. Vaccines are available. Live vaccines should not be used in pregnant ewes or does.
Brucellosis	*Brucellamelitensis* is found around the Mediterranean basin and in the Middle East, Asia and Africa. Abortion storms occur, especially when the bacteria enters a naïve population. There is a live-attenuated vaccine, but this should not be administered to pregnant animals.
Bunyaviruses	Several exist worldwide, including Schmallenberg virus, Akabane virus, Cache Valley fever virus. Spread is by biting insects, and control is based on similar principles to the Schmallenberg virus.
Mycoplasma agalactiae	Found in Southern Europe, Asia, Africa and the Middle East. Clinical signs include fever, corneal inflammation, arthritis, mastitis and abortion. A vaccine is available, which reduces the severity of clinical signs. Other *Mycoplasma* have also been implicated in abortion.
Nairobi sheep disease	A tick-borne viral disease endemic in East and Central Africa. Clinical signs include a high fever, ocular discharges, blood-stained nasal discharges, severe mucoid diarrhoea, dysentery and abortion. Goats are less severely affected than sheep. Vaccination of naïve animals before introduction to an endemic area is recommended. Tick control can help prevent the disease.
Peste des petites ruminants	A contagious viral disease which is seen in sub-Saharan Africa, the Middle East and South Asia. Clinical signs include high fever, nasal catarrh, profuse salivation, profuse foetid diarrhoea, halitosis, pneumonia, and erosions of the mouth, digestive tract and respiratory tract. The nasal and ocular discharges become mucopurulent, and stick the eyelids together and block the nostrils. Abortions occur. A live-attenuated vaccine is available.
Rift valley fever	The virus is mainly found in East Africa, but outbreaks have occurred in Central and West Africa and the Arabian Peninsula. It is spread by mosquitoes. The virus causes hepatitis and vasculitis. Affected animals show fever, jaundice, melaena, diarrhoea, blood-stained mucopurulent nasal discharge and abortion. Deformed lambs or kids may be born. Mortality rates in young lambs and kids may reach 90%. The disease is zoonotic and can be fatal. A live vaccine is available and very effective, giving long-lasting immunity, but should not be used in pregnant animals. A killed vaccine, with a far shorter duration of immunity, is available for use in pregnant animals.
Sheep and goat pox	Found in Africa, Asia and the Middle East. Clinical signs include fever, salivation, nasal discharge and conjunctivitis, and also skin lesions which form vesicles, then pustules, then scabs. Internal lesions in the lungs may lead to respiratory distress. Pregnant adults may abort. Mortality is much higher in lambs and kids.
Wesselbron virus	A mosquito-borne viral disease seen in Southern Africa. It causes abortion in pregnant ewes and does, and may result in the birth of lambs and kids with congenital abnormalities. Neonatal mortality is high, but non-pregnant adults may show few signs other than fever.

Goats are susceptible to all the causes of abortion seen in sheep. Leptospirosis, a relatively common cause of abortion in cattle, has been reported as a cause of abortion in goats. A genetic tendency to abort has been reported in Angora goats. Affected animals tend to be larger than average, and to produce particularly large amounts of fine mohair. They breed successfully as doelings and young does, and the first abortion occurs at 4–5 years of age, at around 100 days of gestation. The dead foetus may be retained for a prolonged period before expulsion. The doe will then cease to carry any foetus to term, and may start to show other abnormalities, such as short oestrous cycles, decreased hair production, muscle wasting and abdominal distension, all due to hyperadrenocorticism.

Managing an Abortion Outbreak

The most effective controls can only be put in place once the cause of abortion has been identified. Nevertheless, several empirical measures can be applied in all abortion outbreaks.

Affected ewes should be isolated as quickly as possible from pregnant sheep and any ewe lambs intended for breeding. They should be kept isolated, ideally until the cause of the abortion is identified, but certainly for at least three weeks.

All products of abortion (placenta, foetuses and fluids) should be collected. If investigation is required, then both the placenta and foetuses should be submitted to a veterinary investigation centre. If not, then they should be buried, if permitted, or burned or bagged and stored safely until collected by a knackery or fallen stock company.

If there is an obvious pattern to the abortion – for example all aborted animals are part of a single group – that group should be isolated and not mixed with other sheep until three weeks after the last animal has lambed. Common sources of feed and water should be inspected.

Individual sick ewes should receive appropriate treatment – for example, oral rehydration solution if dehydrated, antibiotics and anti-inflammatory drugs.

Whole flock antibiotic treatments have been advocated in the face of abortion outbreaks. There is little good evidence to suggest this approach is effective, even with bacterial causes of abortion, and it should not be used as a default response to an abortion outbreak.

Pregnant women, young children, the elderly and immunocompromised people should avoid contact with lambing sheep, especially with aborting ewes and abortion products, due to the high zoonotic risk posed by many of the causes (Figure 5.2).

Identifying the Cause of Abortion

Accurate diagnosis of the cause of abortion can only be achieved through submission of samples to a veterinary investigation laboratory. Certain causes of abortion cause characteristic lesions in either the lamb or the placenta, but these are rarely exclusive to a single cause. The approach to the diagnosis of the cause of abortion depends upon the circumstances in which it is identified.

Ewes that are identified as being barren at the end of lambing time can be blood sampled to identify antibody levels against chlamydial abortion and

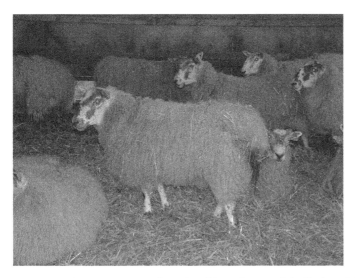

Figure 5.2 Aborted ewes must be isolated from the rest of the flock, and the products of abortion disposed of. Precautions must be taken to avoid the spread of zoonotic infections.

toxoplasmosis. If a large number of ewes is affected, then 5–10 animals should be randomly selected. Interpretation of serological titres can be difficult, but can be made easier if a similar number of ewes which lambed normally are also blood sampled so that the results can be compared.

A vaginal swab can be taken from ewes that are identified as having recently aborted – that is, the presence of blood or birth fluids are seen on the tail, but the foetus or placenta cannot be found. Blood samples can also be taken for serology. Antibody levels are often still rising at the point of abortion, so the most information may be gained by blood sampling 2–3 weeks later. A control group also aids in interpretation. Alternatively, the ewes may be sampled twice, once at the point of lambing and again three weeks later.

The best diagnostic information may be gained from recently aborted ewes by submission of foetus, placenta and a blood sample from the ewe. If cost is a concern, then the foetus and placenta can be submitted, and the blood sample taken later only if no diagnosis is made.

Prevention of Abortion

The prevention of abortion requires a multifaceted approach, given the wide variety of agents that can cause abortion in small ruminants. The risk of causes that are introduced by carrier sheep can be reduced by running a closed flock, or purchasing only male animals. Other agents which are present in the environment, or spread by birds, cats, rodents, or insect vectors, cannot be reliably excluded, though the levels of exposure can be reduced by good management. Vaccines are available against some causes of abortion. Table 5.3 describes common causes of abortion in the UK, and the preventative measures available.

Table 5.3 Preventive measures for the common causes of abortion in ewes in the UK.

Cause of abortion	Preventive measures
Toxoplasma gondii (toxoplasmosis)	Vaccinate. Avoidance of cat faecal contamination of water, feed and bedding is impractical, but keep feed bins secure from cats, and use top bales for cattle. Maintain a healthy population of adult cats on the farm.
Chlamydia abortus (enzootic abortion)	Vaccinate. Maintain a closed flock or source female replacements from accredited free flocks. Lamb bought-in replacements separately in the first year, and investigate all abortions in this group.
Salmonella Montevideo and other salmonella spp.	Maintain a closed flock or lamb replacements separately. Investigate abortions in replacements. Ensure a hygienic environment for late pregnant ewes. Exclude birds and vermin from feed stores. Control vermin. Avoid using troughs, or turn troughs between feeds. Cattle vaccines against *S. Dublin* and *S. typhimurium* may be helpful.
Campylobacter foetus foetus	Maintain a closed flock. Exclude birds from feed stores. Avoid use of feed troughs, or turn and move troughs between feeds. Vaccines are available in some countries.
Broder disease virus	Maintain a closed flock, or test replacement males and females before mixing with the rest of the flock.
Listeriosis	Do not feed spoiled or poorly made silage. Manage the clamp face or big bales correctly. Removed uneaten silage promptly. Minimise soil contamination of silage.
Anaplasmaphagocytophilium (Tick-borne fever)	Introduce potentially naïve replacements early, to ensure exposure to ticks before pregnancy, or keep away from tick pastures until after lambing. Protect against tick bites by organophosphate plunge dipping or pyrethroid pour-ons.
Coxiellaburnettii (Q fever)	Maintain a closed flock. Vaccinate?
Schmallenberg virus	Vaccinate.
Fungi or mycotoxins	Do not feed mouldy or spoiled silage. Store feed correctly. Remove uneaten feed promptly.
Other bacteria	Ensure a hygienic environment for late pregnant and lambing ewes. Move sheep out of muddy poached fields. Avoid feeding spoiled silage.

Diseases of Pregnant Ewes and Does

Identifying problems early is key to successful treatment, and allows timely measures to be put in place to prevent further cases. Animals in the second half of pregnancy should be inspected at least daily and, in the final few weeks of pregnancy, inspection several times a day is recommended. Any ewes or does that do not rise when approached should be restrained and examined. Sick animals often become separated from the rest of the group, so any ewes standing or lying apart from the group should be more closely examined.

Correctly identifying the cause of recumbency, weakness, dullness or unresponsiveness in individual ewes or does is important to ensure that the correct treatment is given, and that appropriate steps to prevent further problems in the flock or herd are taken.

Pregnancy Toxaemia (twin lamb disease)

Ovine pregnancy toxaemia is a result of the increased foetal energy demands in late pregnancy. Ewes mobilise body fat reserves as an alternative energy source when these energy demands outstrip what is available from the diet. If this fat mobilisation is sufficiently large, then it exceeds the capacity of the liver to metabolise the breakdown products. Consequently, the levels of these ketone metabolites in the blood rise, and the liver and kidneys become infiltrated with fat. The clinical signs may reflect the toxic effects of excessive levels of ketones, as well as the acidification of the blood that they cause and the impact of low levels of glucose on brain function. Later in the disease course, animals become dehydrated and develop kidney failure.

Ovine pregnancy toxaemia is commonly seen in thin animals on a poor diet, but is also seen in fat sheep where the diet fails to meet the energy requirements of late pregnancy. It may be precipitated by a stressful event, such as dog worry or bad weather. Ewes carrying multiple foetuses are most at risk.

Affected ewes initially become separated from the group, and may appear dull or unaware of their surroundings (Figure 5.3). They then become blind, although the pupils still respond to light, with fine tremors of the facial muscles. They may be hyper-responsive to stimuli. Affected ewes becomes recumbent as the condition progresses, with decreased abdominal muscle tone, leading to a dropped appearance to the abdomen and making the foetuses easy to feel through the abdominal wall. The condition eventually leads to coma and then death.

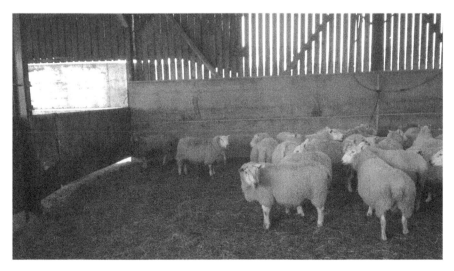

Figure 5.3 A ewe with pregnancy toxaemia has separated from the group and appears unaware of its surroundings.

The clinical signs listed above are often sufficient to make a diagnosis. A blood sample may reveal elevated levels of beta-hydroxybutyrate ketones above 1.1 mmol/l. Ketone levels may also be tested, using urine dipsticks. Elevated urea and creatinine levels indicate renal failure, and suggest a poor prognosis.

Affected ewes which are still able to stand should be housed in a pen alone, with easy access to palatable, high-energy concentrate feed, good quality forage and water. Twice-daily drenching with molasses, propylene glycol or a concentrated glucose-electrolyte drench is advisable. Recumbent ewes have a poorer prognosis, and require intensive nursing if they are to have a chance of recovery. Treatment regimes are often advocated, including the use of propylene glycol or concentrated glucose electrolyte solution drenches, injections of calcium borogluconate, administration of B vitamins, and use of corticosteroid drugs for their anabolic effects. Glucose solution may be given intravenously at the start, but it is rarely cost- or time-effective to maintain blood glucose levels by repeated injections or use of a glucose-saline drip.

As acidosis can develop in the latter stages, the addition of sodium bicarbonate to the intravenous fluids should be considered. Administration of 16 mg dexamethasone by intramuscular injection may induce abortion in some affected ewes after day 136 of pregnancy. A decision to abort the pregnancy should be taken early. A Caesarean section may be considered, as this instantly removes the major energy drain from the ewe. A response to calcium borogluconate injection might indicate the primary problem being hypocalcaemia, and not pregnancy toxaemia.

Recumbent ewes must be bedded and turned regularly, to minimise urine scalding and pressure sores, and also to check for evidence of lambing, as the ewe may be too weak to expel the lambs herself. Fluid intake must be maintained to avoid dehydration and kidney failure.

The prognosis for ovine pregnancy toxaemia is poor, especially once the ewe has become recumbent. Success rates for treatment of recumbent ewes average 30%, though some farmers achieve better than this with very good nursing care. A decision should, therefore, be made early, to humanely euthanise severely affected ewes and to avoid further suffering and compounding of economic losses.

The identification of pregnancy toxaemia in a single ewe should raise concerns for the energy nutritional status of the whole group, and indicates a need to increase the energy density of the ration being fed (Figure 5.4). Increasing the level of concentrate feeding may be counterproductive if it induces ruminal acidosis, consequently lowering the efficiency of forage digestion. It can be helpful to introduce molasses, using ball feeders. Prevention involves ensuring that ewes are in the correct body condition going into the last third of pregnancy. Their diet should be formulated to meet energy requirements, and fed in a manner that allows easy access. Parasite burdens may suppress appetite and also increase energy demands, so should be controlled.

The clinical signs of pregnancy toxaemia in goats are similar to sheep, with the addition of swelling of the distal limbs and tooth-grinding. Fat goats are at particular risk of developing pregnancy toxaemia.

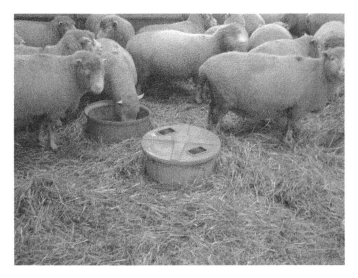

Figure 5.4 Supplementation with molasses using a ball feeder in the face of a pregnancy toxaemia outbreak.

Hypocalcaemia

Hypocalcaemia occurs when the demand for calcium by the growing foetuses is greater than that the ewe can mobilise from her skeleton and obtain from the diet. The disease is often precipitated by sudden stress or feed restriction. It is more commonly seen in older ewes, carrying multiple foetuses, on improved pasture. Calcium is required for muscle activity, so the clinical signs relate to weakness.

Affected ewes are initially separated from the flock due to weakness, and become recumbent. They may initially be able to rise, but tire rapidly and sink back into sternal recumbency. Forestomach turnover ceases, animals become bloated, and passive reflux of ruminal contents may be seen as green froth and fluid around the mouth and nostrils. Affected ewes are constipated, with dry faeces present at the rectum. The body temperature is often subnormal, the heart rate is rapid, and heart sounds and pulses are weak. Affected animals are not blind, but the pupils do not respond to light, or do so only sluggishly. More severely affected animals lie with the head and neck outstretched, and are unable to raise their heads (Figure 5.5).

The clinical signs are usually sufficient to make a diagnosis, but this can be supported by demonstration of serum calcium levels below 1.4 mmol/l.

Most affected ewes respond rapidly to the administration of 20 ml of warmed 40% calcium borogluconate solution, given by very slow intravenous injection. Cold or rapid injection risk causing cardiac arrest. Alternatively, 40–60 ml of warmed 40% calcium borogluconate solution may be given under the skin. Splitting the injection over two or three sites may aid absorption. If diagnosed and treated correctly, then a full recovery may be expected. Relapses do occur, but may be re-treated.

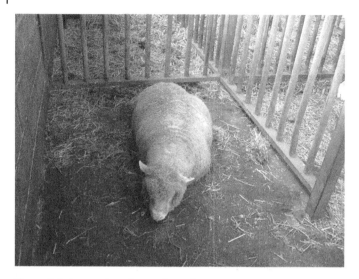

Figure 5.5 A recumbent hypocalcaemic ewe.

The clinical signs and treatment of hypocalcaemia in goats are the same as in sheep. Hypocalcaemia is also seen during lactation in high-yielding dairy goats, usually at 1–3 weeks post-partum.

Ruminal Acidosis (grain overload)

Ruminal acidosis is associated with high levels of concentrate feeding and, hence, occurs commonly in late pregnant ewes. The fermentation of digestible carbohydrates to organic acids decreases the pH of the rumen. This:

i) decreases the numbers of bacteria which produce the volatile fatty acids used by ruminants as an energy source;
ii) increases the number of lactic acid-producing bacteria; and
iii) reduces the numbers of protozoa and fungi, which are necessary for the digestion of long fibre and complex carbohydrates.

Thus, failure to adapt to increased levels of concentrate feed decreases the function of the rumen and levels of energy available to the sheep. If the production of lactic acid is high, for example due to consumption of a large amount of concentrate at one time, then clinical signs of ruminal acidosis will result.

The clinical signs of ruminal acidosis relate to dehydration caused by water being drawn out of the circulation into the rumen due to the high acid concentration, and to a drop in blood pH due to absorption of lactic acid. Affected sheep are dull, depressed, and may be recumbent (Figure 5.6). The forestomach activity is decreased or absent, and bloat may be present. The rumen may lack tone, and feel fluid-filled on palpation. The heart rate is elevated, and the eyes may be sunken due to dehydration. A sour-smelling diarrhoea, sometimes with undigested grains, may be present. Tooth-grinding may occur.

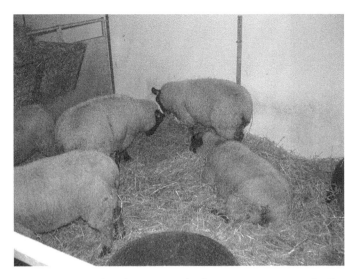

Figure 5.6 Ruminal acidosis as a result of excessive concentrate feeding.

The clinical signs alone may be insufficient to differentiate ruminal acidosis from other causes of depression and recumbency in late pregnant ewes. The history of feeding of high levels of concentrates, or sudden increases in the levels of feeding, aids the diagnosis.

Treatment involves correction of the ruminal acidosis and dehydration. This includes passing a stomach tube, and drenching affected sheep with either a proprietary antacid mixture or with 15 ml of milk of magnesia and 2–4 litres of water every four hours. Intravenous administration of 3–5 litres of isotonic saline spiked with 16 g of sodium bicarbonate is helpful, but the cost may be prohibitive for most cases. A five-day course of penicillin following correction of the acidosis is recommended, to counteract any potential spread of bacteria that have crossed the damaged rumen wall.

Prevention depends on ensuring that the diet is correctly formulated. No more than 60% of the diet on a dry matter basis should be concentrate feed, and ideally no more than 50%. Increases in concentrate feeding should be made gradually, and divided into at least two feeds per day. Feeding should be managed in such a fashion that gorging by individual sheep is prevented. Accidental access of sheep to feed stores should be guarded against.

Hypomagnesaemia (staggers)

Magnesium is vital for the correct function of nerves and muscular tissue. The uptake of calcium is also affected by magnesium absorption. Clinical signs of hypomagnesaemia usually occur following stressful conditions. Magnesium levels in spring grass can be low, but most cases of hypomagnesaemia in sheep are associated with low sodium intakes, which impair magnesium absorption.

Affected animals initially appear nervous and hyperresponsive to stimuli, and have a jerky and exaggerated gait. Muscle tremors may be seen. The disease

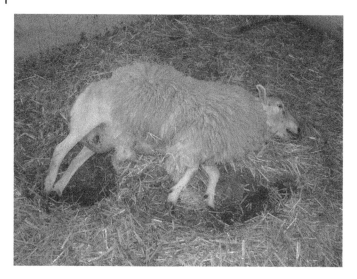

Figure 5.7 Hypomagnesaemia is just one of several differential diagnoses when presented with a recumbent, fitting ewe. The list of other differential diagnoses includes listeriosis and polioencephalomalacia.

progresses rapidly to the animal lying in lateral recumbency, with paddling movements of the limbs and seizures when stimulated (Figure 5.7). The heart rate is elevated, and the heart sounds are increased in intensity.

It can be difficult to differentiate between hypomagnesaemia, cerebrocortical necrosis and listeriosis on the basis of advanced clinical signs alone. The diagnosis of hypomagnesaemia is supported by low blood magnesium levels. A sample of aqueous humour can be taken from dead ewes for magnesium assay.

Treatment of hypomagnesaemia involves subcutaneous injection of 30–60 ml of magnesium sulphate solution. Magnesium sulphate should never be administered intravenously, as this may cause cardiac arrest.

Where outbreaks of hypomagnesaemia occur, it is advisable to ensure adequate sodium intakes by providing access to salt licks. The ration should contain sufficient forage to ensure rumination as a means of recycling sodium-rich saliva and co-transport of sodium and magnesium at the site of absorption in the forestomach. Magnesium supplementation may be given in minerals, lick buckets, water supply or by top-dressing pasture.

Metabolic profiles may include a measure of blood magnesium levels, and can give an indication that intakes are inadequate. Uneven magnesium levels across the sampled group suggest uneven feed intakes, while low magnesium levels across the group suggest a dietary deficit in magnesium.

Cerebrocortical Necrosis (polioencephalomalacia)

Cerebrocortical necrosis may be seen in sheep at any age, but is often associated with over-consumption of rapidly fermentable carbohydrate or very lush grass; hence, it is seen in pregnant and lactating ewes. A lack of vitamin B_1 (thiamine)

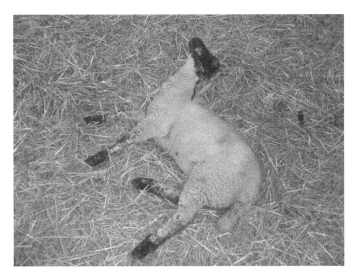

Figure 5.8 A lamb with clinical signs of polioencephalomalacia. The clinical signs seen in ewes are similar.

results in swelling and necrosis of the superficial layers of the brain. Vitamin B_1 is usually produced by bacteria within the rumen, but ruminal acidosis results in a decrease in thiamine-producing bacteria, and an increase in thiamine-degrading bacteria.

Early in the disease course, affected sheep become blind, but their pupils still respond to light. Affected animals are have a high head carriage and are easily startled (Figure 5.8). Head pressing may occur. The pupils are rotated up and towards the nose (strabismus), and spontaneous, repeated lateral eye movements (nystagmus) may occur. The gait may become jerky and exaggerated. More severely affected animals become hyperaesthetic, recumbent, with their head pulled up and backwards, and develop signs of paddling and seizures.

The diagnosis of cerebrocortical necrosis is based on the clinical signs, and supported by a history of increased concentrate intake or movement onto lush grazing. Outbreaks in lambs have been reported following worming. Blood sampling for vitamin B_1 levels, or sampling rumen fluid for thiaminase enzyme levels, can help to confirm the diagnosis, but these are rarely used. On post-mortem, the brain is swollen, and the accumulation of a pigment called lipofuscin within the cortex gives a yellow discolouration and fluoresces under ultraviolet light on the surface of the cerebrum.

Treatment involves injection of 10 mg/kg every 12 hours of vitamin B_1, with the first dose given intravenously. 1 mg/kg of dexamethasone may be given at the first treatment, to reduce brain swelling. If affected animals are treated early enough, they frequently resume eating within 24 hours, although the blindness can take longer to resolve. Affected animals should be housed in a quiet, well-bedded pen, with feed and water within easy reach.

Listeriosis

Listeriosis is caused by the bacterium *Listeria monocytogenes*, which is present in soil and spoiled silage. Consequently, listeriosis is most commonly seen when ewes are being fed silage. The bacteria enters the body through abrasions on the inside of the mouth, or through breaks in the gum caused by the eruption of teeth, and ascends along cranial nerves to the brain, where it causes the development of micro-abscesses.

Affected sheep often have paralysis of one half of the face. There may be deviation of the muzzle, food packing into the cheek, drooling of saliva and drooping of an ear or eyelid. Animals may be dull and may show a propulsive tendency, walking forward before being stopped by an obstacle, or they may circle. The head may be deviated to one side. There is a weakness of limbs on one side of the body, with increased limb extension on the other side (Figure 5.9). In later stages, animals enter lateral recumbency and may show paddling.

The clinical signs and a history of silage feeding can be highly suggestive of a diagnosis of listeriosis. Definitive diagnosis involves the demonstration of microabscessation and *L. monocytogenes* bacteria in the brain at post-mortem examination.

L. monocytogenes is susceptible to a wide range of antibiotics, including penicillin, oxytetracycline and sulphonamide drugs. Twice-daily treatments with high doses of penicillin can be effective. The administration of 1 mg/kg dexamethasone once may be beneficial, but risks inducing parturition after day 136 of pregnancy. Good nursing care is vital. Once animals enter lateral recumbency, the prognosis is very poor.

L. monocytogenes levels are highest in poorly fermented and spoiled silage. Ensuring that only good quality silage is fed to sheep, and that uneaten silage is removed daily, rather than being allowed to spoil, is important.

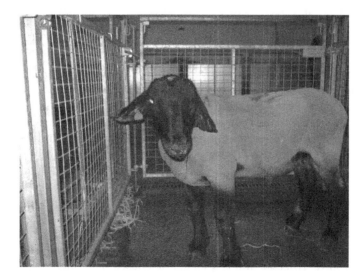

Figure 5.9 A ewe with paralysis of one half of the head, typical of listeriosis.

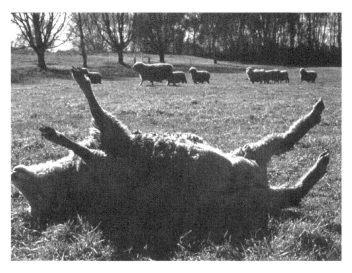

Figure 5.10 Lactating ewes with long fleeces commonly become stuck on their backs, especially after rainfall on warm days.

Ewes Stuck on Their Backs

It is common for individual late pregnant or full-fleeced lactating ewes to become stuck on their backs (Figure 5.10). Certain breeds, over-fat ewes, and those carrying multiple foetuses, are most at risk. When stuck on their back, the weight of the abdominal contents presses on the diaphragm, compromising breathing. Eructation is prevented, so the rumen increases further in size. Ewes that are stuck on their backs are vulnerable to predation or being pecked by corvid birds. While preventing ewes becoming over-fat and managing ectoparasitic infections will help reduce the risk, there is little else that can be done to prevent this occurring. Regular inspection of late pregnant and lactating ewes will allow such animals to be identified and turned right side up in good time.

Downer Ewes

Ewes which have been recumbent for prolonged periods – for example, due to metabolic and infectious disease, or being trapped under heavy snow – develop secondary problems that prevent them from rising once the primary problem has been resolved. Muscle and nerve damage can develop, especially if the ewes are not lying on a well-bedded surface. General weakness can develop due to dehydration and poor feed intakes. Urine scalding and pressure sores may also develop.

Ewes which lie in lateral recumbency should be turned regularly. Food and water intakes should be encouraged, by placing both within easy reach of the ewe. Dehydrated animals can be given glucose and electrolyte oral rehydration solutions by stomach tube. Frequent manipulation of the limbs of downer ewes can help ensure that muscle and nerve function is preserved as far as possible.

Suspending the animal in a sling, such as a feed sack with leg holes cut in it, for 10–20 minute periods several times a day, can also help with a return to weight-bearing and walking.

Vaginal Prolapse

Prolapse of the vagina presents as the eversion and protrusion of the vagina through the vulva (Figure 5.11). The normal mucosal lining of the vagina is smooth, pink and moist but, once exposed, it is prone to damage and may become dirty, abraded or discoloured. The cervix may also be exposed, and seen as overlapping folds of tissue around a central orifice. Affected ewes show signs of discomfort, especially as the prolapse of the vagina kinks the urethra, preventing urination and causing the bladder to become over-full and the ewe to strain. Prolapsed tissue is prone to damage (Figure 5.12), so it should be protected by covering with a damp towel or cloth if it is necessary to move the affected ewe.

Small vaginal prolapses may be gently cleaned, and replaced using pressure with the palms of the hand. Fingers should not be used, as this may tear the vagina. The application of obstetrical lubricant to the exposed lining may aid in replacement. A harness may then be placed on the ewe, to apply pressure to the vulva and back to prevent re-prolapse and reduce the power of straining

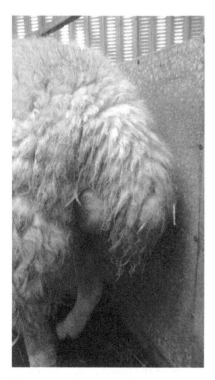

Figure 5.11 A vaginal prolapse in a ewe.

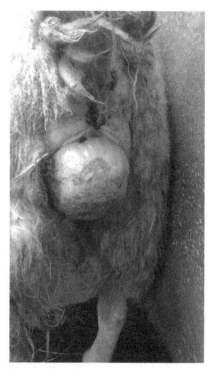

Figure 5.12 Vaginal prolapses are easily traumatised.

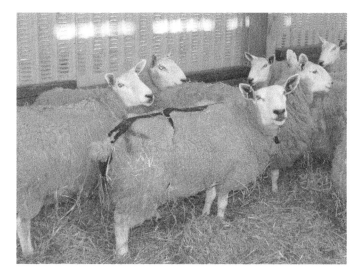

Figure 5.13 Correctly fitted harnesses can be helpful in retaining vaginal prolapses and preventing further straining.

(Figure 5.13). T-shaped plastic spoon devices inserted into the vagina should be avoided, as they can introduce infection and cause further straining.

Larger prolapses, and those where the ewe is straining repeatedly, are best replaced under sacrococcygeal epidural anaesthetic, and restrained using a purse-string suture. Administration of epidural anaesthesia in the UK can only be performed by a veterinary surgeon. Injection to the sacrococcygeal site of 1.8 ml of 2% lignocaine plus 0.2 ml of 2% xylazine gives rapid onset and prolonged duration of anaesthesia. After administration of the epidural, the prolapse is cleaned, lubricated and gently replaced. Elevating the prolapse prior to replacing it may un-kink the urethra, allowing urination and further reducing straining.

Once the prolapse has been replaced, a purse-string nylon tape suture should be placed under the skin around the vulva, to retain the prolapse. This is performed by threading a length of clean 6 mm obstetric tape onto a large curved or half-curved large cutting needle. The needle is inserted into the perineal tissue one finger's width above the bottom of the vulva, at the margin of the haired and hairless skin. The needle then exits at a level midway between the top of the vulva and the anus, and the needle is re-inserted and directed horizontally to emerge at the equivalent point on the opposite side of the perineum. It is then inserted to run vertically, emerging opposite to the first entry point, so that the suture material forms two long sides and one short side of a rectangle around the vulva. The suture is then pulled tight, allowing that a single finger can still be inserted into the vagina.

Tying the suture material in a bow allows it to be undone to check the ewe, if appropriate, and then retied as required. Care should be taken that the suture does not penetrate the vaginal or anal mucosa, as this will lead to infection and thus increase straining (Figure 5.14). Thin or dirty suture materials must not be used, as they will tear out or cause irritation and infection. Other suture patterns,

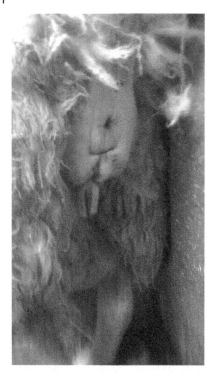

Figure 5.14 Retention of a vaginal prolapse by correct placement of a Buhner suture.

using baler twine or safety pins, are wholly inappropriate.

Ewes with harnesses or retaining sutures should clearly identified, and monitored carefully for the onset of lambing, so that the harness or stitch can be removed. Animals with damage to the vaginal mucosa, or those where sutures are used to retain the prolapse, should receive a course of antibiotics and anti-inflammatory drug treatment. Animals with vaginal prolapses do not usually re-prolapse after lambing, but are considered at greater risk of prolapsing again in future pregnancies, and so should be culled from the flock.

While most ewes which prolapse complete pregnancy and parturition with no further problems, ascending infection from contamination of the prolapsed cervix sometimes leads to death of the lambs and uterine infection.

The likelihood of recovery is very low where the vaginal wall is torn, with the subsequent evisceration of the intestines, or where large areas of the prolapse are cold and discoloured. A decision must be made immediately to euthanise affected ewes in these situations, to prevent further suffering.

Some ewes may prolapse while lambing (Figure 5.15). This may be identified by the observation of protrusion of foetal membranes through the undilated cervix. While replacement of these prolapses is possible, manual dilation of the cervix is often unsuccessful, and the best results are obtained by timely Caesarean section.

Large numbers of vaginal prolapses sometimes occur in certain flocks. Putative risk factors are shown in Table 5.4. It should be emphasised that none of these is proven and, in most cases, the problem has multifactorial causes.

Rectal Prolapse

Prolapse of the rectum through the anus sometimes accompanies vaginal prolapse (Figure 5.16). The exposed rectal mucosal lining is prone to damage.

Small rectal prolapses may be cleaned, lubricated and replaced. If re-prolapse occurs, then a retaining purse string suture may be placed around the anus, under epidural anaesthesia. If the prolapse is damaged or cannot be replaced, then veterinary surgical amputation or repair may be needed. Alternatively, prompt euthanasia may be necessary.

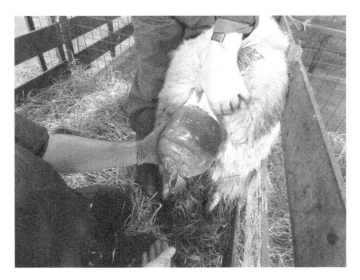

Figure 5.15 The appearance of foetal fluids or membranes through a vaginal prolapse indicates that the ewe is in second stage labour. Most cases require Caesarean section.

Table 5.4 Putative risk factors for vaginal prolapse in ewes.

Tails docked too short
Fat body condition
Multiple foetus pregnancies
Ruminal acidosis
Hypocalcaemia
Bulky feeds
Steeply sloping fields
Insufficient exercise
Crowding and insufficient feed space
Severe coughing

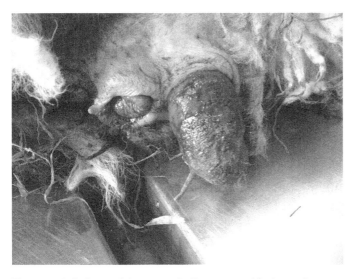

Figure 5.16 Prolapse of the rectum indicates a need for immediate treatment to avoid further suffering.

Prepubic Tendon Rupture

Rupture of the prepubic tendon occurs in older multigravid ewes during the final 2–3 weeks of pregnancy (Figure 5.17). The problem appears to be particularly common in large Half-bred ewes, and is characterised by distinct swelling of the lower left abdomen, immediately cranial to the pubis. In most cases, this leads to rupture of the left ventral body wall, with extensive oedema and displacement of the gravid uterus (Figure 5.18). In some cases, the skin touches the ground and becomes damaged.

Ewes with rupture of the prepubic tendon often have difficulty moving and feeding, leading to pregnancy toxaemia. Affected ewes require close supervision and, in most cases, lambing must be assisted, due to the altered position of the

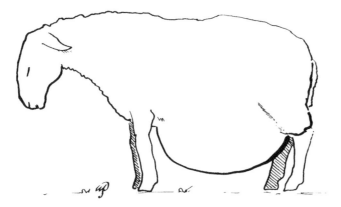

Figure 5.17 A ewe with rupture of the pre pubic tendon (ventral hernia).

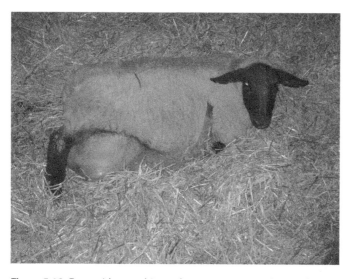

Figure 5.18 Ewes with prepubic tendon rupture are predisposed to pregnancy toxaemia and usually require assistance at lambing.

uterus in relation to the pelvic inlet. Euthanasia is required for welfare reasons, whenever the skin becomes seriously excoriated, the ewe develops pregnancy toxaemia or, sometimes, following delivery of the lambs.

Problems Associated With Pregnancy Occurring After Lambing

Uterine Prolapse

Uterine prolapse results from prolonged and powerful abdominal straining, usually associated with large single lambs and unskilfully assisted lambings. Uterine prolapse may occur almost immediately after lambing, or after an interval of 12–48 hours (Figure 5.19). Those occurring after an interval of 12–48 hours generally result from straining, caused by pain arising from vaginal infection and swelling.

Cases of uterine prolapse require urgent attention to prevent subsequent problems associated with shock, trauma or toxaemia. The principles of replacement are similar to those for the management of vaginal prolapse. Unless the uterus is replaced correctly, and fully inverted to its normal position within the abdomen, the ewe will continue to strain, causing considerable distress and suffering, and will re-prolapse.

Antibiotics should be administered for three to five consecutive days after replacement of the uterine prolapse, to limit bacterial infection of the

Figure 5.19 Uterine prolapse is life threatening and requires immediate skilled attention.

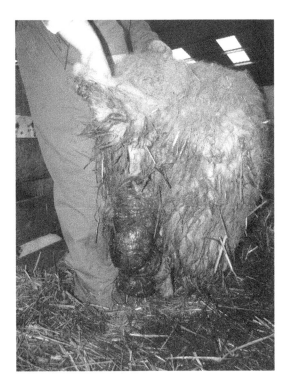

traumatised tissues. The ewe's milk yield will be reduced for a number of days after replacement of the uterine prolapse, and her lambs will require supplementary feeding.

Unlike vaginal prolapse, it is unusual for a ewe to prolapse the uterus the following year, so there is no necessity to cull surviving ewes prematurely.

Uterine Infection (metritis)

Infection of the uterus is seen in ewes after unskilled or unhygienic interference at lambing, after delivery of dead lambs, and following some infectious causes of abortion. Metritis is also common, following replacement of a uterine prolapse.

The diagnosis of metritis is based on the history of dystocia and the exclusion of other diseases of the postpartum ewe. Affected ewes are depressed and inappetant, spend long periods lying down, and show little interest in their lambs. Mucous membranes are congested, and rectal temperature sometimes marginally elevated. The vulva is usually swollen and oedematous, with a red/brown, sometimes purulent, discharge (Figure 5.20). Milk production is poor, and lambs appear gaunt and hungry, attempting to suck whenever the ewe stands.

The response to parenteral antibiotic and soluble corticosteroid treatment is generally good. Failure to respond to treatment indicates the presence of a retained foetus, or a concurrent disease such as mastitis or peritonitis associated with uterine rupture.

Clostridial infections sometimes occur 1–3 days after difficult and unhygienic lambings. The disease is characterised by marked swelling of the vulval and perineal areas, oozing of blood-tinged droplets from the vulval wall and adjacent skin, and dark red areas of necrosis extending to adjacent muscles.

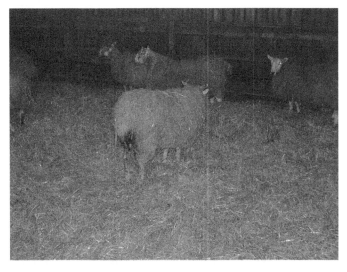

Figure 5.20 A dark coloured discharge and sick, depressed ewe signals metritis, requiring immediate treatment.

The risk of metritis can be greatly reduced if unnecessary interference with lambing ewes is avoided, great care is taken not to injure the reproductive tract of lambing ewes, and simple hygienic measures are adopted for all assisted lambings. These measures should include washing hands and lambing aids in antiseptic solution, the use of clean disposable arm-length plastic gloves, use of obstetrical lubricant, and judicious use of long-acting antibiotics following assisted lambings. In multigravid litters, delivering only the lamb in malpresentation or malposture, rather than all of the lambs in quick succession, greatly increases the likelihood of introducing infection deep into the uterus.

Kangaroo Gait

Kangaroo gait is probably a metabolic disease. It is usually seen in inadequately fed ewes suckling twin lambs, but the cause is unknown. Affected sheep remain bright and alert, but show difficulty in placing their forelimbs, sometimes knuckling at both front fetlocks, and move with shortened strides, with their pelvic limbs drawn well forward under the body, propelling them forward with a characteristic bounding gait (Figure 5.21). Most affected animals recover spontaneously after their lambs are weaned. Important differential diagnoses include vertebral abscessation, elbow arthritis and any painful condition affecting both forefeet.

Mastitis

Mastitis causes substantial economic losses and welfare concerns associated with ewe deaths, reduced lamb growth rates, perinatal lamb mortality and involuntary culling of chronically affected animals.

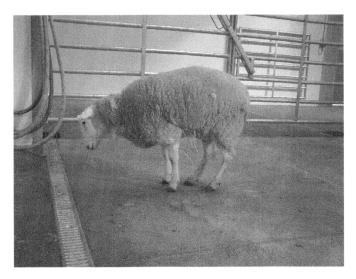

Figure 5.21 The cause of kangaroo gait is unknown, but it is thought to be a metabolic disorder arising at lambing.

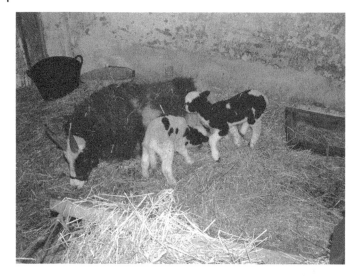

Figure 5.22 A recumbent ewe with a hot and painful udder and hungry lambs, indicative of acute mastitis.

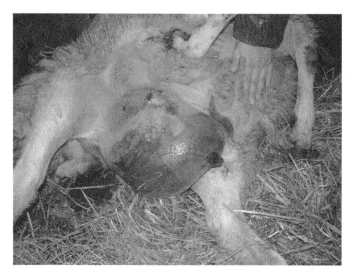

Figure 5.23 In cases of acute mastitis, the udder is initially hot and painful, rapidly becoming cold and purple-coloured.

Most cases of acute mastitis are seen within three weeks of lambing (Figure 5.22). Most flocks experience an annual incidence of about 2% but, in many, the incidence is considerably higher. Affected ewes do not feed, and often appear lame in one hind limb. The udder is initially swollen, hard, warm and painful, but may become cold and purple-coloured within a few hours (Figure 5.23). Many ewes die as a result of generalised toxaemia. Those that survive are generally ill thrifty, and the affected side of the udder eventually sloughs, to reveal finger-like protrusions of deeper glandular tissue. These often become secondarily infected and fly-struck.

Early cases respond well to macrolide antibiotic treatment. However, the treatment response is poor where the udder is already cold, purple-coloured and gangrenous, in which case ewes should be euthanised, to avoid further suffering and ill thrift associated with chronic suppurative infection. Those that survive are usually emaciated by the time of weaning.

In less severe cases, the udder does not become cold and necrotic, but abscesses form within the tissues as the acute infection subsides. Subsequent milk yields are reduced, and lamb growth rates and weaning weights are poor. Chronic mastitis may go unrecognised during the initial stages of the disease, but is later identified by the presence of hard swellings within the udder. These cases are often not detected at the time of weaning, when ewes are still lactating, but are found after the subsequent lambing, when milk production is poor. In problem flocks, ewes' udders should, therefore, be re-checked before mating.

Mastitis in lactating ewes usually results from bacterial infection of the udder by bacteria normally present on the skin of the teats or in the tonsils of young lambs. Mastitis occurs when these bacteria have the opportunity to enter into the normally protective teat canal. This can occur when the ewes' milk supply is insufficient, resulting in excessive suckling by lambs and teat injury. Lesions on the teats, poor udder conformation, poor mothering behaviour, or exposure of the teats to cold winds, can also predispose to mastitis. Occasionally other opportunistic bacterial pathogens are involved, associated with a wet, dirty environment, or with dirty hands checking newly lambed ewes for milk flow.

Prevention of acute mastitis depends on identifying the predisposing factors. In most cases, the underlying cause is poor milk production, which can be addressed in subsequent years by attention to the body condition and protein nutrition of ewes during the second half of pregnancy. There is some evidence to support the use of dry cow mastitis tubes or macrolide injections in problem flocks at weaning, but substantial data are not available to determine the cost-effectiveness of these strategies. Furthermore, administering whole-flock prophylactic antibiotic treatments may be shown to be irresponsible with reference to selection for antimicrobial drug resistance. Furthermore, unless mastitis tubes are infused under strict hygienic conditions, their use may prove counter-productive.

Induction of Abortion and Parturition

Foetal maturation in sheep and goats occurs very late in gestation, hence induction of parturition usually results in the birth of nonviable offspring unless this occurs very close to the date of parturition. Consequently induction of parturition is occasionally used to abort undesired pregnancy due to mis-mating, or in the management of pregnancy toxaemia, but has little role in tightening the lambing period. Regimes that can be used to induce abortion or parturition in sheep are shown in Table 5.5.

Table 5.5 Induction of abortion or parturition in ewes.

Drug	Dose	Timing of treatment	Hours to parturition or abortion	Notes
PHF2α or analogues	Varies with precise product	<30 days	Too early in gestation for abortion to be observed	After day 30, this method is unreliable as the placenta produces progesterone.
Betamethasone	10 mg	141 days	45 ± 15	Use of corticosteroids will lead to some degree of foetal maturation.
Dexamethasone	10–20 mg	140 days	42 ± 7	
Dexamethasone	1.5 mg	146 days	69 ± 7	
Flumethasone	2 mg	140 days	44 ± 14	
Cloprostenol	0.0375 mg	146 days	104 ± 18	High risk of lack of foetal maturation. Increased risk of retained foetal membranes.
Cloprostenol + dexamethasone	1.5 mg + 0.0375 mg	143 days + 144 days	68 ± 14	Increased risk of retained foetal membranes.

Table 5.6 Induction of abortion or parturition in does.

Drug	Dose	Timing of treatment	Hours to parturition / abortion	Notes
PHF2α	2.5–5 mg	7–10 days after buck removed.	Too early in gestation for abortion to be observed.	Care must be taken, as some of these does will come back into oestrus 48 hours after treatment, and so are at risk of being mated again. Increased risk of retained foetal membranes.
Cloprostenol	125–150 μg	From five days after buck removed.	Too early in gestation for abortion to be observed.	
Dexamethasone	10–20 mg	144 days	48–72	Use of corticosteroids will lead to some degree of foetal maturation.
Flumethasone	2 mg	144 days	48–72	
PHF2α	15 mg	143 days	36–60	PHF2α/analogues can be used earlier in pregnancy than this, but there is a very high risk, if used earlier, that the kid will not be viable.
Cloprostenol	125–150 μg	143 days		

Unlike ewes, female goats are reliant on the corpus luteum as the source of progesterone to maintain pregnancy throughout gestation. Thus, prostaglandin F2a or its analogues can be used to terminate pregnancy at any point. Regimes that can be used to induce abortion or parturition in does are shown in Table 5.6.

6

Identifying Unwell Ewes and Lambs, Does and Kids

Ewes and Does

Normal Behaviour

The first step to successful treatment of any sick individual is the early identification of any problems. It is necessary to understand the normal appearance and behaviour of ewes, does, lambs and kids, as a basis to identify the presence of abnormalities. It can be helpful to compare animals with possible abnormalities with their healthy, normal flock or herd mates.

Sheep are flock animals and will usually move as part of the group. Any animal which is separate from the rest of the group is acting abnormally, and should be investigated. At pasture, sheep spend the majority of their time actively grazing, or lying and chewing the cud. Animals do not usually stand idly. The majority of sheep managed under commercial conditions regard humans as predators, and will move away if approached closely. The flight response will vary with the degree of human contact the sheep are accustomed to, as well as the breed, the age of the animal (ewe lambs and gimmers are often flightier) and between individuals. Sheep do not usually permit a close approach.

Itching (pruritus) and rubbing behaviour may occur with a variety of diseases. Severe pruritus – for example, seen with sheep scab and scrapie – is such that animals are not easily distracted from these behaviours, unlike with milder pruritic diseases (for example, louse infestation). Severely pruritic animals may show a reflex whereby rubbing the back results in a nibbling movement of the lips, and may even precipitate seizure-like events.

Due to the way they tend to be managed, a greater proportion of goats are tolerant of close approach by humans. They are also intrinsically more curious than sheep, and will use their mouths to investigate novel items in their environment. Goats are also much more vocal and less stoic than sheep, and will bleat loudly in protest at procedures which would not cause obvious discomfort from a sheep.

Goats climb frequently, with consequent injuries. They also are not deterred by barbed wire, and so it should not be used for fencing goat paddocks, otherwise injuries may result. If using a post and rail or a strainer system for fencing, these should slope inwards, otherwise goats will climb up them. They are also capable of undoing simple latches.

Practical Lambing and Lamb Care – A Veterinary Guide, Fourth Edition.
Neil Sargison, James Patrick Crilly and Andrew Hopker.
© 2018 John Wiley & Sons Ltd. Published 2018 by John Wiley & Sons Ltd.

When threatened, goats tend to face the threat and make a characteristic sneezing noise. Goats' tails usually point up unless sick or distressed. Pruritic goats will rub against solid objects, but will also turn and bite and chew at their own coat.

Signs of Inflammation

Most infections or injuries result in inflammation. Inflammation has four main signs:

  i) redness;
 ii) swelling;
iii) heat; and
 iv) pain.

Body Condition

Several methods have been developed to assess and score the body condition of sheep (described in Chapter 3). The most commonly used with reference to targets for different stages of the production cycle employs a five-point scale, from 1 (emaciated) to 5 (obese).

Where all, or the majority, of the sheep in a group are too thin, possible causes include inadequate quality, quantity or access to nutrition, or a widespread disease problem, such as liver fluke or haemonchosis. Where a smaller number of animals are in poor body condition, this will relate to individual circumstances – for example, ewes carrying multiple foetuses, individual animals being bullied away from the feed face, lameness, tooth problems, or slow onset infectious diseases.

Goats store more of their body fat within the abdomen, so the body condition scoring system for sheep cannot be directly applied to goats. However, the principles of target condition at each stage of the production cycle are the same as for sheep.

Observation of the Head

When sheep are not grazing, drinking or investigating an object, their head is usually carried level with, or above, the withers, although the precise mode of head carriage varies with breed, due to different body shapes. Abnormally low head carriage may indicate neck pain or a neurological problem. Extension of the neck often accompanies respiratory disease as the animal tries to increase air intake with each breath. Tilting of the head or deviation of the nose to either flank may indicate a brain lesion.

Ear carriage varies with breed. For example, Suffolks have drooping ears and Border Leicesters have pricked ears, but these should be symmetrical. A single drooping ear may indicate facial paralysis, as seen in listeriosis. Ears may become swollen due to injury or infection. Sick sheep often have symmetrically drooping ears.

The eyes should appear bright and alert. Any discharge from the eyes is abnormal. Cloudiness of the cornea (the front of the eye) is often the first sign of eye infection. Other signs include frequent blinking, discharge, and the appearance of small blood vessels in the front of the eye.

Eye position should be symmetrical, and the eyes should move when the head is moved. Abnormal eye positions suggest a neurological problem.

The ability of the eye to detect light may be tested by shining a light into the eye (this is best performed out of direct daylight). The pupil should shrink in response to the light. A sluggish or absent response of the pupils to light may indicate damage to the eye or optic nerve, or hypocalcaemia (as this leads to weakness of the muscles of the iris and slows nerve conduction).

Blindness is detected using the menace response, where a finger is rapidly brought close to the eye and the animal should blink. Failure to blink indicates blindness (although, if the test is repeated many times, the sheep may become used to it and cease blinking).

The ocular aperture (the opening between the eyelids) should be symmetrical. Asymmetry often occurs with eye injury or nerve injuries. Normal sheep have wide ocular apertures when awake (the exception is while lying and chewing the cud). Reduction in the size of the ocular aperture, for example by partial lowering of the upper eyelid, is a very sensitive and early indicator of pain or illness.

A very small amount of clear, watery nasal discharge is normal. Larger amounts of discharge, especially if the discharge is thick or cloudy, indicate a problem of the respiratory tract. Discharge from one nostril usually indicates the problem is located in the nose. Problems further down the respiratory tract usually produce discharge from both nostrils. The air flow from the nostrils can be tested by holding a bare hand in front of each nostril in turn and should be equal.

Inspection of the incisor teeth can be performed simply by folding down the lower lip. Checking the cheek teeth is more difficult but palpating along the outside of the mandible (jaw bone) for any swellings can identify problems. The cheek teeth are very sharp, so a hand should never be placed into a sheep or goat's mouth.

Tooth problems may also lead to packing of food into the cheek, causing a bulge, drooling of saliva, often staining the chin green-brown, and the dropping of partially chewed bits of food. Such signs may also been seen with facial paralysis or tongue injuries.

The corner of the sheep's mouth turns up slightly. Loss of this appearance occurs when the cheek muscles are tightened, as occurs in pain or illness.

The face should be symmetrical. The symmetry may be disrupted by swellings such as bruising, tumours, cheek packing, or deviation due to paralysis. Tremors and twitches often occur with metabolic problems, such as pregnancy toxaemia and hypocalcaemia.

Facial changes in goats in response to examination and illness are the same as in sheep. Goats carry their head above the level of the withers, unless eating or drinking. In addition to the facial structures shared with sheep, goats may also have wattles hanging below the mandible. These structures contain blood vessels, nerves and smooth muscle around a cartilaginous core, and occasionally become swollen due to the development of wattle cysts. Scent glands are found in bucks in the skin behind the horns but, unlike sheep, goats do not have scent glands below the eye.

Mucous Membranes

Mucous membranes line the body cavities. They can be inspected in the mouth, the inside of the eyelids and the third eyelid, and also the inside of the vulva. The normal colour in sheep is pale pink, but those in the mouth may be melanin-pigmented. Various changes to mucous membrane colour occur, making good indicators of various disease states.

Pale-to-white mucous membranes indicate a paucity of supply of red blood cells to the periphery. This may be due to low red blood cell levels (anaemia is commonly caused by haemonchosis or liver fluke infection), low blood volume (hypovolaemia), perhaps due to rapid blood loss or severe dehydration, or heart failure.

Reddening of the mucous membranes indicates that the blood vessels have become dilated, causing (distended) injected or congested mucous membranes, as occurs during systemic infections. Local inflammation will also cause reddening – for example, infection in one eye will cause reddening of that eye's mucous membranes. A diffuse dark red colour occurs during kidney failure.

During severe infections, toxins are released from the bacteria causing the infection. This, in turn, has an effect on the circulatory system causing stasis and pooling of blood in the smallest blood vessels (capillaries). This results in a congested appearance of the mucous membranes, eventually proceeding to a purple discolouration, especially around the base of the incisor teeth. These changes indicate severe disease.

Other mucous membrane colour changes may occur with rarer disease states – for example, jaundice associated with the breakdown of red blood cells during copper toxicity. Focal bleeding may be seen in the mucous membranes as red specks, due to problems with blood clotting.

Observation of Breathing

Sheep pant to cool down and when stressed, so breathing rate is not a good indicator of respiratory disease. Increased breathing effort, as denoted by larger movements of the ribs, flaring of the nostrils and increased abdominal breathing movements, are better indicators of respiratory problems. Abnormal respiratory noises such as rasping, roaring, whistling or crackling, which can be heard without a stethoscope, indicate severe respiratory disease.

Movement

Sheep should be able to move freely, with even strides. Lameness is indicated by the carrying of a foot when standing or walking, head-nodding, obvious limping, an uneven stride length and a tendency to kneel to graze.

Weakness may manifest as scuffing of toes. This is often more easily heard on a hard surface than seen.

Neurological problems may result in the paralysis of a limb, causing it to be carried or for the foot to be placed incorrectly. They may also cause weakness, a swaying gait with abnormal step placement (ataxia), or abnormal behaviours such as circling, leaning on walls or fences, or a progressive tendency, where the animal moves aimlessly forwards before encountering an obstacle, at which point it stops.

Tremors are usually seen with metabolic problems.

Lameness in goats manifests itself similarly to sheep. Marked swelling of the carpus often occurs with caprine arthritis and encephalitis (CAE).

The interdigital space, between the two toes, may be lightly haired. The skin should be intact, and there should be no unpleasant smell. The two most common foot problems of sheep and goats – scald and foot rot – cause reddening of the interdigital skin and the development of a grey scum. With foot rot there is also a characteristic smell.

The hoof walls should be tightly adhered to the coronary band at the top. Separation of the hoof walls occurs in both foot rot, where the separation commences at the interdigital space, and in contagious ovine digital dermatitis (CODD), where the separation commences on the outside of the foot, usually at the front. The separation in both diseases may extend down the wall, under the sole and up the other hoof wall. A discharging tract at the coronary band indicates a hoof abscess under the wall.

The hoof wall should be tightly joined to the sole horn at the white line. Separation and packing of the resultant space is referred to as 'shelly hoof', and may progress to abscessation, or may result in lameness in its own right.

The length of the hoof walls is not usually itself a cause of lameness, and overly long hoof walls associated with lameness are more often a consequence of reduced wear, rather than a cause. Trimming of hoof horn in cases of foot rot and CODD is to be discouraged, as it slows down healing and may help to spread the infection through contamination of hoof shears.

Protruding, pink, fleshy growths (granulomas) surrounded by loose horn, usually at the toe, may be seen. These result from exposure and irritation of the soft tissue beneath the hoof horn (corium), due to over-trimming or untreated foot rot.

A variety of bacterial and viral infections may cause lesions around the coronary band. Blisters (vesicles) could be a sign of foot-and-mouth disease, which is notifiable. Proliferative fleshy lesions result from infection with the orf virus (which is zoonotic, so such lesions should be handled only with gloves on).

Swelling of the foot above the coronary band and severe lameness is associated with joint infection of the pedal joint.

Goats are also affected by foot rot and scald. CODD-like lesions have been described, as have erosive lesions which begin at the sole or white line. Goats overfed on concentrates develop inflammation of the layer which attaches the hoof capsule to the rest of the foot (laminitis). This presents as a symmetrical lameness, and affected animals often have very thick, hard soles, due to the abnormal horn produced. Goats that are kept on soft bedding, with limited opportunities for exercise on a hard surface, may develop overgrown feet, as the hoof horn grows faster than it is worn down. Corrective trimming may be required in these cases.

There is a scent gland above the interdigital space in sheep (but not in goats), which usually contains a small amount of grey, waxy substance. If this contains pus, or the surrounding area is hot, swollen or painful, this indicates infection of this gland.

Lame animals where no cause can be found in the foot should have their legs carefully palpated. Joint swelling may result from infection or injury. Chronic arthritis of a joint results in new bone formation around the joint.

Fractures of the lower limb are often obvious because of deviation of the line of the limb and lameness, due to the animal's avoidance of putting weight on the affected limb. Higher in the limb, the fracture may be detected by careful palpation of the leg. There is usually marked swelling around the fracture site. Consideration must be given to the fact that palpation of the fracture is painful.

Observation of the Abdomen

Small changes in abdominal shape are hard to assess in sheep which have full fleeces. The forestomach occupies the left flank. An animal which has not been eating for several days will have a hollow appearance to the flank on this side. By contrast, an animal with gas trapped within the rumen, causing bloat, will have a bulge high on the left flank. The lower abdomen will enlarge in late pregnancy, due to the increase in the size of the uterus. Very enlarged abdomens may indicate a problem with the uterus or gut.

The line of the underside of the abdomen should be a smooth curve, from the groin region forwards. A steep bulge may indicate rupture of the pre-pubic tendon or the abdominal wall.

The Fleece or Coat

The appearance of the fleece gives a general indication of the health of the animal. In sheep, animals suffering from chronic malnutrition, trace element deficiencies or chronic disease, will have poorer quality fleeces. Fleeces of unhealthy ewes may appear open, or the crimp may be reduced and the wool fibres easily broken.

Animals which have suffered a severe disease event or nutritional stress and have then recovered may shed parts of their fleece, due to a break in the wool. The underlying skin should appear healthy, and the regrowth of wool should begin almost immediately.

Tags of wool protruding from the fleece may indicate mild pruritic disease, as described earlier. Bare patches with damaged skin indicate more severe pruritus. Sheep scab also causes the oozing (exudation) of serum fluid onto the skin. This dries into characteristic scabs, beneath which may be seen the very small, pearly white mites.

Goats in poor health may have a dull coat, with hair loss and a scurfy appearance.

Observation of the Breech

Soiling of the fleece of the tail and breech region with faeces indicates diarrhoea. A foul-smelling, red-brown discharge from the vulva after lambing is an indication of uterine infection.

Swelling of the vulva with oedema, but no other changes, may occur pre-lambing, but usually resolves after lambing. A swollen vulva, with discolouration, exudation of fluid and a cool, clammy feel indicates clostridial infection of the tissue (gangrene).

Faecal soiling due to diarrhoea in goats is more commonly noted on the hocks. Goats have scent glands beneath their tail, and a waxy, brown secretion in this area is normal.

Examination of the Udder

The udder increases in size during the final few weeks of pregnancy, and becomes filled with the colostrum (first milk), which is thick and yellow. The normal udder is warm to the touch, and the skin is dry and pliable.

Heat, reddening and swelling of the udder, along with clots or blood in the milk (which may become watery or yellow) are all indications of mastitis. In cases of gangrenous mastitis, the udder skin becomes purple, and then blue or black, and is cold and clammy to the touch. Ewes affected with mastitis may appear lame from a distance as they walk, to minimise pain from the inflamed udder half. Mild cases of mastitis may present with just changes to the milk secretion, but without obvious signs of udder inflammation or systemic illness.

Occasionally, small blood vessels rupture within the udder, to give a pink tinge to otherwise normal milk. Such animals do not require any treatment, as the problem is self-resolving.

Chronic cases of mastitis present with lumps within the udder, which should not be confused with the normal plates of secretory tissue – one within each half of the udder. Tracts discharging pus from abscesses may be seen, and the affected half may appear empty, as its milk-producing activity has been reduced.

Lambs and Kids

Normal Behaviour

Normal lambs, when roused from lying, will stand, stretch and then move freely. Lambs over several days of age will show a variety of play behaviours, such as jumping and racing with other lambs. Normal lambs will suck vigorously once the teat is located, and will shake their tails during this process and butt the udder to stimulate milk let-down. Lambs which are reluctant to stand, or stand hunched, are lame or do not suckle vigorously, merit further inspection.

Goat kids are as fond of play as lambs. While lambs tend to accompany their mother everywhere, gradually expanding the distance from her that they are prepared to roam, the behaviour of goats is different. Does will leave kids camped in a safe concealed place, and then return every 2–8 hours. As a doe needs to know the geography of an area well to be able to find her kids again, they should not be moved to new enclosures just before kidding.

Neonatal Lamb Behaviour

Immediately after birth, the lamb usually raises its head and shakes it vigorously several times before commencing breathing efforts. Vocalisations follow after five minutes, and the lamb usually attempts to stand within 15 minutes. The ewe stimulates the lamb by vigorous licking. Ewes may strike out at, or nudge, unresponsive lambs with a forefoot. Lambs will usually suckle within an hour of birth. They locate the udder by looking at the junction of the horizontal line of the belly and the vertical line of the hindlimb and, hence, lambs may end up misdirected to the oxter, or may struggle to find the teat, in ewes with very pendulous udders.

Ewe-lamb bonding occurs within the first 6–12 hours of life. If the lamb is removed during this time, the ewe will reject it when it is returned.

Identifying Feed Intake

Good colostrum intake within the first hours of life is vital to lambs, both in terms of the acquisition of immunity, and as an energy source. Lambs which have suckled well can be identified by the fuller appearance of their abdomen, when compared to those that have not suckled well, which have an empty or hollow appearance to the abdomen. This can be appreciated most clearly if the lamb is picked up by the front legs and the abdomen gently palpated.

Watery mouth disease causes gut stasis, and so affected lambs often appear to have a full abdomen. However, as their distended abomasum contains much gas as well as fluid, a sloshing or rattling sound is heard if the lamb is picked up.

Abnormalities More Commonly Seen in Lambs Than Adult Sheep

As indicated, many of the abnormalities of body systems described for ewes above also pertain to lambs. However certain changes or findings are more frequently encountered in lambs.

Milk appearing at the nostrils indicates a split hard palate. Such lambs will not be able to suckle or feed effectively, and should be euthanised.

In-turned eyelids (entropion) are seen commonly in lambs and should be corrected as soon as detected, to avoid secondary damage to the eye.

Bleeds of the oral and ocular mucous membranes may indicate a prolonged birth. Such lambs are likely to take longer to stand and suckle, and require closer attention.

Swelling (oedema) of the head is often seen following head-only malpresentation dystocias. The oedema resolves after lambing, but these lambs may take longer to suckle.

Rib fractures along the edge of the sternum can occur when too large a lamb has been delivered vaginally, or if assistance has been rough or unskilled. The fractures may be seen as an indentation of the lower part of the chest wall. Fractures higher on the ribs also occur. Limb fractures are also seen in lambs. They usually occur when the ewe treads on the lamb, or if the lamb gets the limb trapped in a gate, fence or hurdle. There is usually a very good response to casting or splinting, depending upon the site of the fracture.

Abdominal distension may be caused by atresia ani, where the anus does not have an external opening and so the lamb cannot defecate and, consequently, becomes bloated due to trapped faecal matter. Such cases are often not noticed until several days have passed. The condition can sometimes be successfully remedied with a simple operation, provided that other internal abnormalities are not present.

The normal faeces of milk-fed lambs are yellow and are often soft or pasty in consistency in the neonatal period. When diarrhoea occurs, it is mostly seen as faecal staining on the perineum and hocks.

Rectal Temperature

Body temperature is elevated during systemic infectious disease, but then falls again in cases of severe disease. Body temperature may also be elevated due to environmental effects or vigorous activity on the part of the animal.

The normal body temperature range of adult sheep is 38.8–40.0 °C. The normal temperature range of goats is 38.6–40.6 °C.

7

Legislation

This chapter covers the aspects of UK legislation which deal with issues of animal welfare and national infectious disease control that are likely to be encountered during the pregnancy and parturition of sheep and goats. The principles that are described are relevant globally.

The full scope of the legislation is not given. Some legislation varies between the devolved administrations of the UK and legislation in other countries may be very different. Legislation also changes over time, so it is, therefore, necessary to check for up-to-date information from the correct sources. Within the UK, the Department for Farming and Rural Affairs (DEFRA), or the relevant body in the devolved governments or administrations, should be contacted for clarification.

Welfare Legislation

Keepers of animals have a legal obligation to ensure the welfare of their animals. The guiding principles behind the current welfare legislation can be summarised as five freedoms:

  i) freedom from hunger and thirst;
 ii) freedom from discomfort;
iii) freedom from pain, injury and disease;
 iv) freedom to express normal behaviour;
  v) freedom from fear and distress.

Various other definitions of animal welfare may be applicable in some circumstances and forums, but they are underpinned by the aforementioned five freedoms.

Codes of Recommendations

Various pieces of legislation govern the codes of recommendations for the welfare of livestock. These summarise the duties of keepers with reference to the welfare of their animals. Following the guidance contained in these codes will

Practical Lambing and Lamb Care – A Veterinary Guide, Fourth Edition.
Neil Sargison, James Patrick Crilly and Andrew Hopker.
© 2018 John Wiley & Sons Ltd. Published 2018 by John Wiley & Sons Ltd.

ensure that animal keepers do not break the law. Failure to observe code recommendations could be used as evidence to establish guilt in cases where animal suffering is identified. All keepers should have access to, and an awareness of, the codes for the relevant species.

The code of recommendations for sheep is freely available online as a.pdf: https://www.gov.uk/government/uploads/system/uploads/attachment_data/file/69365/pb5162-sheep-041028.pdf (accessed April 2016).

The code of recommendations for goats has not yet been put into booklet format, but is available here: http://adlib.everysite.co.uk/adlib/defra/content.aspx?id=000IL3890W.16NTBXIX24U1AI (accessed April 2016).

The quality of stockmanship is the single most significant influence on the welfare of the flock or herd. If the shepherd or goatherd is over-worked, inexperienced or under-skilled, then animal welfare will suffer. Relevant extracts from the code of recommendations for the welfare of sheep, first published in August 2000, are shown in Table 7.1.

Acts of Veterinary Surgery

Acts of veterinary surgery may only be performed by veterinary surgeons. For anyone else to perform them is illegal.

Opening any body cavity is considered to be an act of veterinary surgery, as is disbudding of goat kids or lambs, dehorning, vasectomy, and use of an electro-ejaculator for semen collection as part of a breeding soundness examination.

Castration of lambs and goat kids may be performed by competent lay people over the age of 18 years, but only on animals below three and two months of age, respectively.

Mutilations

Tail-docking and castration are mutilations and, no matter which method is used, there is a degree of short-term and long-term pain associated. Consequently, if these procedures can be avoided by good management, this option should be taken wherever possible. Castration should only be performed if lambs will be kept past puberty and separate management of males is not possible.

Tail-docking may only be performed where there is considered to be a high risk of tail soiling and fly strike. Most tail-docking is performed by the application of a tight rubber ring to the tail. The regulations governing this are:

i) this may only be performed on animals not more than seven days old;
ii) use of an anaesthetic is not mandatory;
iii) the tail must be docked such that it is long enough to cover the vulva of females and the anus of males.

Castration should only be performed if lambs will be kept past puberty, and separate management of males is not possible. Castration should only be performed after the ewe/lamb or doe/kid bond has formed. Lambs and kids are

Table 7.1 Extracts from the Code of Recommendations for the Welfare of Livestock: Sheep (as summarised in the 3rd Edition of this book).

Health

(20) Stockmen should be experienced and competent in the prevention and treatment of foot rot, the techniques of lambing, injection and oral dosing, tail docking and castration of lambs. It is particularly important that shepherds have competence in the skills required at lambing time.

(21) A written health and welfare programme for all animals (including pregnant ewes, lambs and breeding replacements) should be prepared for each flock. This should cover the yearly production cycle. It should be developed with appropriate veterinary and technical advice, and reviewed and updated annually. The programme should include sufficient records (including lambing records) to assess the basic output of the flock, and should address, as a minimum, vaccination policy and timing and control of external and internal parasites and foot care.

(25) The health and welfare of animals depends upon regular supervision. Shepherds should carry out inspections of the flock at intervals appropriate to the circumstances in which sheep are kept, and pay particular attention to signs of injury, distress, illness or infestation, so that these conditions can be recognised and dealt with promptly. The frequency of inspection will depend on factors which affect sheep welfare at any particular time, such as housing, lambing, fly strike and adverse winter weather conditions.

(32) Where external parasites are likely to occur, such as those causing scab or fly strike, ticks or lice, sheep should be protected by dipping, or by the use of an effective preventive chemical agent. Where sheep are clinically infected with such external parasites, effective treatment must be given without delay.

(33) Internal parasites should be controlled by grazing management and/or anthelmintic treatment, administered at appropriate times, based upon the life cycle of the parasite. Advice on appropriate timing and steps to avoid the development of anthelmintic-resistant worms should be sought from a veterinary surgeon or specialist adviser.

Casualties

(34) Injured, ailing or distressed sheep should be identified and treated without delay. Where the shepherd is able to identify the cause of ill health, he or she should take immediate remedial action. When in doubt, veterinary advice should be obtained as soon as possible.

(35) Provision should be made for the segregation and care of seriously sick and injured animals. Unfit sheep should be removed from flocks.

(36) If an unfit sheep does not respond to treatment, it should be culled or humanely killed on farm. It is an offence to cause, or to allow, unnecessary pain or unnecessary distress, by leaving a sheep to suffer.

(37) In an emergency, it may be necessary to kill an animal immediately to prevent suffering. In such cases, the animal should be destroyed in a humane manner and, where possible, by a person experienced and/or trained both in the techniques and the equipment used for killing sheep.

Dosing and vaccination

(40) Special care should be taken to ensure that all equipment used in dosing, vaccination and treatment is maintained to a satisfactory standard. Equipment used for any injection technique should be frequently cleansed and sterilised, to avoid infections at the site of injection. Disposable needles should be used whenever possible. Needles and dosing gun nozzles should be of a suitable size for the age of the sheep. Hazardous objects such as needles should be disposed of safely, in accordance with current legislation.

(Continued)

Table 7.1 (Continued)

Management

(58)
Castration   Farmers and shepherds should consider carefully whether castrating within a particular flock is necessary. Castration is unlikely to be necessary where lambs will be finished and sent to slaughter before reaching sexual maturity. Account should be taken, not only of the pain and distress caused by castration, but also the stress imposed by gathering and handling and the potential risk of infection. Castration should not be performed until the ewe-lamb bond has become established. Castration must be carried out only in strict accordance with the law, and by a competent and trained operator.

(62)
Tail docking   Farmers and shepherds should consider carefully whether tail docking within a particular flock is necessary. Tail docking may be carried out only if failure to do so would lead to subsequent welfare problems because of dirty tails and potential fly strike. If it is considered that both tail docking and castration are necessary, thought should be given to performing both operations at once, to minimise disruption and the potential for mis-mothering and distress. Tail docking must be carried out in strict accordance with the law.

Pregnancy and lambing

(72)   The nutritional management of pregnant ewes is particularly important. Both condition scoring and ultrasound scanning, to determine the numbers of foetuses present, will be of benefit in assessing dietary needs.

(73)   Pregnant and nursing ewes should receive sufficient food to ensure the development of healthy lambs, and to maintain the health and bodily condition of the ewe.

(75)   Heavily pregnant ewes should be handled with care, to avoid distress and injury that may result in premature lambing.

(76)   Severe damage and suffering can be caused through inexperience when assisting a ewe in lambing difficulties. Shepherds should, therefore, be experienced and competent before having responsibility for a flock at lambing time. Where necessary, they should receive proper training in lambing techniques.

(77)   Stockmen should pay particular attention to cleanliness and hygiene. Every effort should be made to prevent the build-up and spread of infection, by ensuring the lambing pens are provided with adequate clean bedding and are regularly cleansed and disinfected. It is particularly important to ensure that dead lambs and afterbirth are removed and disposed of by incineration, without delay. Lambing pens, sufficient in size and number (i.e. one pen per eight ewes, or one pen per four ewes where synchronised mating is practised), should be easily accessible on a dry, well-drained site. Each pen should be provided with a hay rack, feed trough and water bucket. If the pens are outside, the tops should be covered.

    There is a potential health risk to pregnant women from aborting ewes, ewes at risk of abortion, dead lambs and afterbirths. Pregnant women should stay away from sheep at lambing time.

(78)   There may be times when even a proficient shepherd experiences difficulty in delivering a lamb single-handed. In such cases, assistance should be called immediately.

(79)   Any ewe with a prolapse should be treated immediately, using an appropriate technique. Where necessary, veterinary advice should be sought.

(82)   Stockmen should be trained in resuscitation techniques and survival aids, such as feeding by stomach tube and use of a warmer box.

(83)   It is vital that every newly born lamb receives colostrum from its dam, or from another source, as soon as possible and, in any case, within three hours of birth. Adequate supplies of colostrum should always be stored for emergencies.

Table 7.1 (Continued)

(85)	Where lambing takes place out of doors, some form of (natural or artificial) shelter or windbreak should be available.
(86)	The problems of mis-mothering, which occur particularly during gathering, handling, transport or dipping of ewes and lambs, should be reduced by keeping group size to a minimum. Careful marking of lambs and mothers may also be beneficial, using non-toxic colour markers.
(87)	Wherever possible, young lambs should never be sold at market unless they are with their mothers. Arrangements should be made for direct transfer of orphan lambs between farms, rather than through markets, to minimise disease risks. It is illegal to transport, and offer for sale at market, lambs with an unhealed navel.

Artificial rearing

(88)	Artificial rearing requires close attention to detail and high standards of supervision and stockmanship to be successful. It is essential that, where possible, the lambs should be allowed to suck the ewe for at least the first 12 hours of life.
(89)	All lambs should receive an adequate amount of suitable liquid food, such as ewe milk replacer, at regular intervals each day, for at least the first four weeks of life.
(90)	From the second week of life, lambs should also have access to palatable and nutritious solid food (including grass), and should always have access to fresh, clean water.
(91)	Where automatic feeding equipment is provided, lambs should be trained in its use, to ensure an adequate intake of food. The equipment should be checked daily to see that it is working properly.
(92)	Troughs should be kept clean, and any stale food removed. Equipment and utensils used for liquid feeding should be thoroughly cleansed at regular and frequent intervals, and should be effectively sterilised.
(93)	A dry bed and adequate draught-free ventilation should be provided at all times. Where necessary, arrangements should be made to provide safe supplementary heating for very young lambs.
(95)	Suitable accommodation should be available for sick or injured lambs. This should be separate from other livestock.
(96)	Until weaning, housed lambs should be kept in small groups, to facilitate inspection and limit the spread of disease.
(97)	Where young lambs are being reared at pasture without their mother, care should be taken to ensure that they have adequate shelter.

Buildings and equipment

(107)	Floors should be designed, constructed and maintained so as to avoid discomfort, distress or injury to the sheep. Regular maintenance is essential. Solid floors should be well-drained and provided with some form of dry bedding. Newly born and young lambs should not be put on slatted floors unless suitable bedding is provided.
(110)	Water bowls and troughs should be constructed and sited so as to avoid fouling, and to minimise the risk of water freezing in cold weather. They should be kept thoroughly clean, and should be checked at least once daily, and more frequently in extreme conditions, to ensure that they are in working order.
(111)	Troughs should be designed and installed in a way that will ensure that small lambs cannot get into them and drown.

(Continued)

Table 7.1 (Continued)

(112)	For sheep given concentrate feed, when all animals are fed together, it is important to have adequate trough space to avoid competition and aggression. In normal practice, approximately 30 cm of trough space is needed for hill ewes, and approximately 45 cm for the larger lowland ewes. Excessive competition is detrimental to sheep welfare. Over-crowding may lead to increased incidence of prolapses.
(113)	When feeding hay and silage *ad libitum*, trough space should normally be 10–12 cm per ewe, dependent upon size. Racks and troughs should be positioned and designed to avoid injury, discomfort and damage to sheep.
	Safe feed-trough design is particularly important for housed lambs who, like children, love exploring, and appear to have an unrivalled ability for getting themselves trapped in all sorts of awkward areas! Broken limbs, crush injuries or worse have become more common in recent years, largely due to the increased popularity of feeding big bale silage, or hay that occasionally topples over inside the feeder.

Lighting

(114)	The law requires that fixed or portable lighting should be available, so that sheep kept in buildings can be thoroughly inspected at any time.
(115)	Throughout the hours of daylight, the level of indoor lighting, natural or artificial, should be such that all housed sheep can be seen clearly.

Space allowances

(116)	The space allowance and group size for housed sheep should be determined according to age, size and class of livestock. The minimum feed space for hill breeds weighing 40–60 kg, for *ad lib* forage and concentrates, is 10 cm and 30 cm respectively. The minimum feed space for lowland breeds weighing 60–90 kg, for *ad lib* forage and concentrates, is 12 cm and 45 cm respectively. More feed space is recommended for horned sheep, or those carrying more than two foetuses. The minimum lying space for pregnant lowland ewes weighing 60–90 kg, pregnant hill ewes weighing 45–60 kg, lowland ewes with lambs at foot, hill ewes with lambs at foot and rams is 1.2–1.4, 1.0–1.2, 2.0–2.2, 1.8–2.0 and 1.5–2.0 m^2, respectively.

Hazards

(127)	Young lambs should be protected, as far as is possible, from hazards such as open drains and predators.

most frequently castrated by application of a tight rubber ring at the neck of the scrotum. This may only be performed on animals not more than seven days old; however, an anaesthetic is not necessary.

Surgical castration may be performed without anaesthetic before three months old (two months in goats), but lay persons performing this must discuss it with their veterinary surgeon first. Surgical castration after three months old (two months in goats) is an act of veterinary surgery.

While not frequently performed, the removal of supernumerary teats may be required in milking sheep or goats. Specific legislation does not exist but, extrapolating from cattle legislation, use of an anaesthetic should be mandatory if the animal is over three months old.

Disbudding and dehorning of goats and sheep is an act of veterinary surgery, and may only be performed by a vet. Anaesthesia is mandatory. Disbudding of goat kids should be carried out before they are ten days old. Removal of the insensitive tip of a growing horn, where otherwise it will impinge on the animal's face or head, may be performed by lay persons.

Illegal Procedures

The following procedures are illegal, and should never be carried out under any circumstances:

i) penile amputations or any other penile operation;
ii) the procedure referred to as tooth grinding;
iii) electro-immobilisation;
iv) freeze dagging.

Transport

Animals should not be transported in such a way that is likely to cause injury or unnecessary suffering. Animals which are ill, injured, infirm or fatigued should not be transported. Lambs and kids should not be transported before their navel is completely healed. Lambs and kids under one week old should not be transported more than 100 km. Pregnant ewes and does should not be transported after 90% of gestation has passed (after approximately 130 days of pregnancy), or within one week of giving birth.

There is an exemption to these rules, in that animals may be transported to veterinary premises for treatment, even if they would ordinarily be excluded from transport. For example, a new-born lamb with a broken leg may be transported to a veterinary surgery for treatment. However, all steps must be taken to prevent unnecessary suffering during transport – for example, the lamb's leg should be splinted if possible, and the lamb confined in a cardboard box to prevent it being thrown around the vehicle during transport.

Euthanasia

If required, euthanasia must be performed in a timely and humane fashion, by an appropriately skilled person. Appropriate methods of killing adult sheep and goats include shooting, captive-bolt stunning followed by exsanguination, or inserting a rod into the brainstem (pithing), and injection of barbiturates (legislation surrounding on farm slaughter for human consumption will not be covered here).

Freely available information on shooting and captive bolt stunning may be found on the Humane Slaughter Association website: www.hsa.org.uk (accessed April 2016).

When shooting sheep or goats with a free bullet, it is important that this is done safely. Firearms should not be discharged in such a way that the bullet could strike a person if it passes through the animal in question. To minimise the risk of ricochet, the firearm should not be discharged towards a wall or solid floor, and great care must be taken if using the weapon inside a building.

Humane killers (specifically adapted single-shot weapons) and shotguns are the most appropriate firearms. 0.22 rim-fire rifles may be used, but these can be extremely dangerous if the point of aim is wrong. Larger calibre rifles are inappropriate for use in close-quarters for euthanising sheep or goats, and should be avoided. Humane killers are used in full contact with the animal's head, while shotguns and 0.22 rifles should never be placed in contact with the animal's head, but should be aimed with the muzzle 5–25 cm from the animal's head. No. 4, 5 or 6 bird shot is appropriate for use in shotguns for euthanasia. Round-nosed lead bullets should be used with rifles or humane killers. All local legislation regarding the licensing and keeping of firearms must be obeyed.

The point of aim for all firearms in polled sheep (those without horns) and goats is a point in the midline of the face, just above the eyes, with the line of fire down the spine into the upper body (Figure 7.1). In heavily horned sheep and goats, an alternative point of aim, just behind the poll, with the line of fire directed down the axis of the head, may be used with a shotgun, provided the animal is standing on soft ground.

A captive bolt stunner uses percussive force to render the animal unconscious (Figure 7.2). It must then be killed by another method. Captive bolt stunners may be non-penetrative or penetrative. If the animal is to be killed by bleeding out, either type may be used.

The point of aim for the captive bolt in polled sheep is the highest point of the skull, aiming straight down (Figure 7.3). In horned sheep, the point of aim is on the midline, behind the ridge connecting the horns, aiming towards the base of the tongue (Figure 7.4). The point of aim in all goats is behind the bony mass on top of the skull, which lies between the horns in horned goats on the midline, aiming towards the base of the tongue.

Immediately following stunning, the neck should be severed, using a sharp knife with a blade at least 120 mm long, just behind the angle of the jaw. The cut should reach from ear to ear, be deep enough that it reaches the spine, and should sever

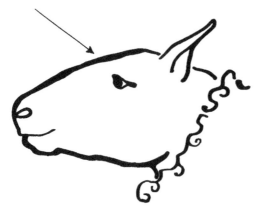

Figure 7.1 Aiming position for a shotgun in young or polled animals or free bullet weapon in adult animals.

Figure 7.2 A captive bolt pistol with cartridges used to propel the bolt. The apparatus must be well maintained after use.

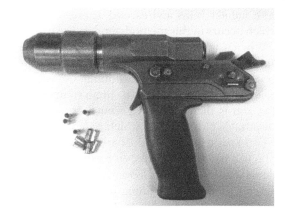

Figure 7.3 Aiming position for using a captive bolt in young or polled animals.

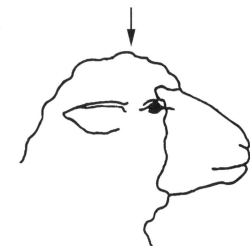

Figure 7.4 Aiming position for using a shotgun or captive bolt in older or horned animals.

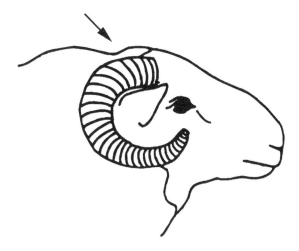

both jugular veins and carotid arteries. Severing the oesophagus and trachea, which occurs in this method, renders the carcase unfit for human consumption.

When using a penetrative captive bolt stunner, which makes a hole in the skull, pithing by use of a wire or rod to destroy the brain may be used, rather than exsanguination. Following stunning, the wire or rod should be inserted into the hole and directed towards the brain stem and spinal cord at the back of the skull. The rod is then moved vigorously back and forth, to destroy the brain stem. Disposable pithing canes which remain in the carcase are available.

Euthanasia by injection of barbiturates is available only to veterinary surgeons, who will have been trained to carry out the procedure in a humane and professional way. Injection of an overdose of barbiturate anaesthetic will result in death. Several products containing pentobarbitone are available on the market. The recommended dose rate is 150 mg/kg. Barbiturates are extremely irritant if administered extravascularly, so care must be taken that the needle is well within the vein. The jugular vein is most commonly used. This may be raised by applying the fingers of one hand to the transverse processes of the cervical vertebrae, and then moving them towards the midline. The fingers will then obstruct the jugular vein, causing it to fill with blood and raise. At this point, the vein can be located by palpation, or by visualisation in hair sheep, shorn sheep and short-haired goats. The position is quite variable for much of its course, but it has a fixed point at the angle of the jaw. It may be located here and then followed back to an appropriate site for injection. Alternatively, the cephalic vein on the cranial aspect of the forelimb (antebrachium) can be used.

If the animal is very collapsed and it proves impossible to raise a vein, then intracardiac injection is acceptable as a last resort. A long spinal needle will be required to reach the heart in large sheep. The animal is placed in lateral recumbency, the upper most forelimb pulled forward, and the needle inserted perpendicular to the body wall in the area usually covered by the elbow. Barbiturate euthanasia renders the carcase unfit for human consumption.

Appropriate methods of euthanasia for neonatal lambs and kids include injection of barbiturate by a vet, and blunt trauma followed by exsanguination. The latter may be delivered by holding the animal up by the hind legs and delivering a swift, sharp blow to the back of the head using a heavy, blunt object. Alternatively, the blow may be delivered by swinging the lamb or kid's head hard against a wall or other hard object, while holding the lamb by the hind legs. In both cases, the blow must be extremely hard and sure. It should be followed by a cut across the neck just below the angle of the jaw, from ear to ear, to the depth of the spine.

Record Keeping

Sheep and goat keepers are legally obliged to keep a register of animals kept on each holding. The keeper must record in the register: details of new or replacement identifiers applied to sheep or goats; movements to and from the holding; deaths, including the date and identifier (if known); and an inventory of all the sheep and goats on the holding on 1st December each year.

The register may be kept on paper, electronically using any software, or online on the Animal Reporting and Movement Service (ARAMS) website. It must be submitted for inspection as required.

Traceability

The traceability of livestock is vital for the investigation and control of animal diseases on a national level, for the protection of international trade, to ensure confidence in trade of animals within the UK, and for the protection of human health through food safety.

All holdings with any sheep or goats on them in the UK (or any other farmed species other than fewer than 50 poultry) must have a CPH (County Parish Holding) number. This is a nine-digit number which serves as a unique identifier for the holding. The first two digits represent the county, the next three the parish, and the last four the holding. A CPH number is acquired by contacting the Rural Payments Agency.

All sheep and goats must have an official identifier applied to them:

  i) by six months of age if housed overnight;
 ii) by nine months of age if not housed overnight; or
iii) before they leave the holding (at any age).

In an emergency, an unidentified animal may be moved off the holding for veterinary attention, but an identifier must be applied immediately upon its return, and the movement must be recorded in the holding register.

Animals that will be slaughtered before 12 months old may have a single ear tag (slaughter tag) which displays only the herd or flock number. They cannot also have a management tag. Any animal which will be kept beyond the age of 12 months must have two identifiers, which have an individual animal number as well as the herd or flock number.

In animals where only one identifier is required, this must be an ear tag. In animals where two identifiers are required, these may be two ear tags or an ear tag plus one of:

  i) an electronic identification device (EID) bolus;
 ii) a tattoo, usually inside the ear; or
iii) a pastern band, which may be an EID or non-EID.

All sheep must have one electronic identification device under EU law. Goats need not have an EID identification method, but cannot be exported without one. The available EID devices include:

  i) ear tags;
 ii) boluses; and
iii) pastern bands (if this is the EID device the animal cannot be exported).

For goats, there is the additional option of a passive injectable transponder (microchip) inserted under the skin of the groin (if this is the EID device, the animal cannot be exported).

For sheep under 12 months of age, the single slaughter tag must be an EID ear tag, though the tag may display only the flock number. The EID ear tag must be yellow (in England and Wales), and should be inserted into the left ear. EID tags may be any colour in Northern Ireland and Scotland. The EID pastern band must be yellow. If the animal has an EID bolus or pastern band, then the ear tag must be black.

Missing tags must be replaced with 28 days of the loss being noticed. The numbers on the two identifiers must match. With tags, a matching replacement tag can be ordered and applied, or the remaining tag can be removed and a new pair inserted. The second option is not possible with a tattoo, bolus or pastern band.

When an animal originates from outside the EU, any existing ear tags should be removed and a pair of matching red ear tags applied.

Protection of Human Health

There is a statutory obligation on employers to take reasonable steps to protect the health of their employees, by providing a suitable working environment, suitable equipment and relevant training. While this applies all year round, it warrants particular consideration at lambing or kidding time, because:

i)   many causes of abortion in small ruminants are zoonotic;
ii) the level of close contact with sheep and goats and their bodily fluids and waste products is much higher than the rest of the year;
iii) the frequent employment on farm of temporary or casual labour to cope with the increased labour demands; and
iv) the long hours of work at lambing/kidding can cause tiredness, resulting in impaired judgement.

There is, thus, a duty upon farmers to make employees aware of the zoonotic risks, provide appropriate protective equipment such as gloves, and hygiene facilities such as sinks for hand washing, and to ensure that any employees or volunteers who may not be familiar with the farm and sheep or goats are made aware of the hazards inherent in their role, and are trained sufficiently to mitigate these.

Medicines Usage

Sheep and goat keepers must record: the name and address of the supplier of all medicines; the date of treatment; quantity, product and batch number. The identity of treated animals must also be recorded. These records must be kept in writing, and be permanent and available on request. Records and proof of purchase of medicines must be kept for at least five years. Disposal of unused medicines must also be recorded.

Under EU law, all veterinary medicines used in food-producing species must have an established maximum residue limit (MRL). Drugs without an MRL for a food-producing species cannot be used in any food-producing species, regardless of whether the animal is intended for human consumption or not. The full list may be found here: http://ec.europa.eu/health/files/eudralex/vol-5/reg_2010_37/reg_2010_37_en.pdf (accessed April 2016).

In the first instance, the drug chosen should have a license for use in that species and for the treatment of that condition. The dose rate and dosing interval will be displayed on the bottle, as will the withdrawal periods.

The number of licensed products for sheep is limited, and for goats is very low. Where there is no drug licensed for that species and that condition, then a system referred to as the cascade must be followed. The next step is to use a drug licensed for a different condition in that species, or in another food-producing species. If no such suitable drug is available within the UK, then a suitable product may be imported from another EU member state, providing the product is licensed for a food-producing species there. In these circumstances, the prescribing veterinary surgeon must specify an appropriate withdrawal period. It is advised that this must be a minimum of seven days for milk and 28 days for meat, or the withdrawal period for the species for which it is licensed, whichever is longer. The veterinary surgeon responsible for prescribing the product must also keep specified records.

The withdrawal periods for products exist to protect human health from pharmaceutical contamination of foodstuffs. The withdrawal periods of products must be obeyed. Animals must not be sent for slaughter within the meat withdrawal period, and milk must be withheld from the bulk tank for this period. The withdrawal period must be adjusted accordingly where the product is used off-license – for example, in an unlicensed species, at an unlicensed dose rate or frequency, or for an unlicensed treatment period.

Disposal of Waste

Disposal of waste is covered by a variety of legislation, depending on the category of waste. Needless to say, inappropriate disposal of waste threatens human health, animal health and the environment.

Fallen Stock

From a legislative perspective, fallen stock refers to dead livestock, stillborn or aborted foetuses and placentas. Fallen stock cannot be buried or burned. The exception to this includes remote areas (the Isles of Scilly, Lundy Island, Bardsey Island and certain areas of the Scottish highlands and islands) and during natural disasters. While pet animals can be buried, sheep and goats, even if kept as pets, cannot ever be buried.

Table 7.2 Notifiable diseases of sheep and goats in the UK.

Disease	Clinical signs	Zoonotic
Anthrax	Sudden death, dark tarry blood from the mouth, nostrils, vulva and anus.	Yes
Aujesky's disease	Primarily a disease of pigs but, if other species are infected, they become intensely pruritic, scratching even the flesh from their bones. It is inevitably fatal.	
Bluetongue	High fever, abortion, oedema (swelling) of the tongue and muzzle, bleeding or swelling of the coronary band, often fatal in small ruminants.	
Brucellosis (*B. melitensis*)	Abortion storms, fever, depression, mastitis, arthritis, orchitis (infection of the testicles) or nervous signs. Clinical signs may be rare in chronically affected flocks or herds.	Yes
Contagious agalactia	Fever, keratitis (infection of the cornea), arthritis, mastitis, abortion.	
Contagious epididymitis	Fever, depression, epididymitis.	
Foot and mouth disease	High fever, death in young animals, development of vesicles (blisters) in the mouth and around the coronary band. These may then rupture to form ulcers with ragged edges.	
Goat pox	Fever, salivation, nasal discharge, conjunctivitis. Skin lesions which form vesicles, then pustules, then scabs. Internal lesions in the lungs may lead to respiratory distress.	
Peste des petits ruminants	High fever, nasal catarrh, profuse salivation, profuse foetid diarrhoea, halitosis, pneumonia. Erosions of the mouth, digestive tract and respiratory tract. The nasal and ocular discharges become mucopurulent, and stick the eyelids together and block the nostrils.	
Rabies	Mainly affects carnivores, but sheep and goats may be affected. Sudden onset neurological signs and jaw paralysis. Inevitably fatal in all unvaccinated mammals (including humans).	Yes
Rift Valley Fever	Fever, hepatitis (liver infection), abortion storms, very high mortality in neonatal lambs.	Yes
Scrapie	Usually seen in sheep aged 2–5 years old. Insidious onset of clinical signs. Intense pruritus, behavioural changes (aggression, depression), incoordination and weakness, weight loss, death.	
Sheep pox	In lambs, the disease is rapidly fatal. Signs include a high fever, paralysis, and red spots on the membranes of eyes and nose and the wool-free areas of skin. In older sheep, signs include high fever, reduced appetite and spots, as described for lambs, but these may also occur on woolled areas. The spots develop into large, oozing pimples, which then become covered in a crust. Pregnant ewes may abort.	
Tuberculosis	Small ruminants are rarely infected, compared with cattle, deer and camelids. The disease primarily presents as wasting, with enlarged lymph nodes.	Yes

All fallen stock must be collected, identified and transported from the farm as soon as it is reasonably practicable. While awaiting collection, fallen stock should be stored so that animals and birds cannot access the carcase. Fallen stock may be stored in bins, but these must have a lid, be leak-proof and be cleaned and disinfected when empty. It is the farmer's responsibility to arrange the collection of the carcase by an approved transporter, and its transport to:

  i) a knackery or fallen stock recovery service;
 ii) a hunt kennel (animals within the withdrawal period of drugs, or euthanised by barbiturate injection, should not be sent to a hunt kennel);
iii) a maggot farm;
 iv) an incinerator; or
  v) a renderer.

Used hypodermic needles and scalpel blades are considered to be hazardous waste. They must be collected in an appropriate container.

Pharmaceutical products are considered to be hazardous waste. The recommended means of disposal for small quantities of pharmaceuticals, including used vials or bottles, is to return them to the supplier – for example, a veterinary practice or animal health outlet. Local authorities are obliged to collect such waste when asked to so by the waste holder, but it must be kept separately from other waste. A charge may be made to cover the cost of collection.

Notifiable Diseases

Certain diseases which are considered to pose a severe hazard to livestock farming and/or human health are classed as notifiable. Anyone who suspects that an animal has a notifiable disease must notify the Animal and Plant Health Agency (AHPA) immediately. Once a notifiable disease is suspected on a premises, no animals or people should move on or off the holding until notified that it is acceptable to do so by APHA. If a notifiable disease is confirmed on the holding, then all movements will be controlled.

The notifiable diseases affecting sheep and goats (as at date of publication) are shown in Table 7.2.

In Scotland, sheep scab is notifiable. Clinical signs include pruritus, wool loss, the formation of flaking yellow crusts on affected areas of skin, under which the mites may be just visible to the naked eye as pinpoint white specks.

Certain diseases are reportable. In these cases, the disease is reported to APHA by the appropriate laboratory once the disease has been diagnosed. Examples include *Salmonella* and sheep scab in England and Wales.

Index

Practical Lambing and Lamb Care – A Veterinary Guide, Fourth Edition.
Neil Sargison, James Patrick Crilly and Andrew Hopker.
© 2018 John Wiley & Sons Ltd. Published 2018 by John Wiley & Sons Ltd.

Printed and bound by CPI Group (UK) Ltd, Croydon, CR0 4YY

27/10/2024

14580363-0004